Supplemental:

Bridgeport ☐
Bay Path ☐
MassPharm ☑
Albany Med ☑
Stony Brook ☐

An Applicant's Guide to Physician Assistant School and Practice

Second Edition

Erin Sherer

An Applicant's Guide to Physician Assistant School and Practice

Acknowledgments

This book never would have been written without the enthusiasm and foresight of my husband, James. He has always been loyal in his support, and intense in his interest. His creativity, constructive criticism, and diligence in editing truly made this book possible.

I would also like to thank my mother-in-law, Judith Savo, and my father-in-law, Albert Savo, for allowing me to live with them while I worked on this project. Without their constant support and encouragement, this book would not have been updated.

I would like to offer special thanks to my mentor, Dr. Ahmad Hakemi, for his support and for teaching me several valuable lessons—namely about professionalism, hard-work, and the importance of providing students with high-quality education despite the obstacles associated with doing so. I will be forever grateful.

I would like to thank my colleagues in the American Association of Surgical Physician Assistants (and fellow PA educators), Jerry Simons, Robert Blumm, and Robert Sammartano. In addition to being mentors to me for several years, they each spent a great deal of time reviewing the book and providing me with ideas about how to improve it.

I am also indebted to a number of current physician assistants and students who helped make this book even better: David Payne, Alicia Smiley, Gloria Peterson, Jamie Peterson, Amy Marchewka, Thomas O'Brien, Lucas Wyzlic, Erin Werner, and Ashley Froede.

The book cover design was created by an incredibly tech-saavy physician assistant, Alex Corcoran. I am appreciative for his vision and enthusiasm.

Special thanks as well to several of my colleagues who work in physician assistant education and continue to inspire me: Dan Vetrosky, Roy Constantine, Ron Nelson, Rebecca Lowrence, Matthew Stack, John Lopes, Clint Fitzpatrick, Barb McIntyre, William Saltarelli, Matthew Smith, James Lile, Michael Moutsatson, Teresa Ashley, Peggy Clerc, and Kristen Edgerton.

And, finally, I would like to thank my parents, Jan Baker and Chuck Bomba, and my sister, Kristin Bomba, for always supporting me in all of my personal and professional endeavors.

Table of Contents

Introduction

Once upon a time, I was in your shoes. I was considering applying to physician assistant (or "PA") school, but I had little background knowledge about the profession, or about whether or not I might actually be a competitive applicant. Like you, I researched the process. After carefully considering my options, and, using the method I outline in this book, I successfully gained entrance to physician assistant school.

Now, as a practicing PA and educator, I am eager to help those interested in becoming a part of this profession. My goal with this book is simple: I want to help ambitious students gain admission into PA school programs by providing readers with a solid background of the PA profession (how it exists today, and where it is headed tomorrow), and giving readers skills and advice helpful in becoming a successful PA school applicant and future healthcare provider.

As a new physician assistant, it is a daunting task to "learn the ropes" of the profession on your own, on the job. Certainly, during PA school you will figure out some of the basics, but after graduation your professors are no longer guiding you along, or helping you to figure things out. Simply put, you are back in charge.

It is exciting to finish school, but what comes after can be overwhelming and stressful. Becoming certified, finding a job, negotiating a contract, knowing how to bill for your services – these are all things you must do as a practicing PA; however, oftentimes no one teaches you these things in PA school.

I decided to write this book because when I looked back on everything that happened during my journey to becoming a practicing PA, I realized there were many things I struggled with that might have been different with one or two crucial facts, and many of these difficulties happened due to inadequate guidance. I want to share what I have learned with those who are just beginning the process of becoming a PA. Learn from my successes, and from my mistakes—and good luck as you begin your future career in one of the most exciting professions in healthcare.

How to use this book

This book will help guide you along the process of becoming a PA. It begins by helping you, the prospective PA student, consider whether or not you really should become a physician assistant—by discussing what a PA really does, and comparing the PA profession to other healthcare careers. This book provides you with the necessary information to successfully apply to physician assistant educational programs, while also providing tips that will enhance your abilities to interview well, and discuss the PA profession intelligently. Finally, this book includes several indices that will provide you with more information about each accredited PA program in the United States as well as additional resources for students and practicing physician assistants.

Another goal of this book is to help the new PA figure out how to become an organized, knowledgeable, and confident professional. I will guide you along the steps you will take as a newly-minted PA: from graduation, to certification and licensing, to finding a job, to negotiating a contract, all the way to obtaining the appropriate CME to maintaining your credentials as a PA.

The chapters were written with a novice in mind, so if you read the book straight through (even if you have little or no background knowledge of the physician assistant profession), you will have no problem following the concepts. Also, this book is organized into a series of steps which build upon one another, ultimately leading you through PA school, and on to becoming a practicing PA. While some parts of the book are quite general, others will examine specific topics related to the PA profession and the PA school application process.

This book is primarily patterned after my own experience, but I have tried to provide concrete examples both from my own experiences working in the profession, as well as examples from other practicing clinicians. These examples will give you accurate and realistic ideas about your PA application and eventual PA practice within the profession. While some chapters may initially seem superfluous, each is important, and may help a prospective student or practicing PA when he or she least expects it. Ideally, you should read this book in its entirety before you begin applying to PA school, and use it as a reference during PA school and beyond.

Be advised, this book is not guaranteed to help you gain admission to PA school. Unfortunately, there is no magic formula to gaining PA school admission. That being said, by reading this book and researching the profession before you apply, you are starting off on the right foot.

I hope you find this book to be both useful and enjoyable, and I wish you the best of luck as you begin your journey to successfully becoming a physician assistant.

Part I: About the PA Profession

What is a Physician Assistant?

We should begin with the basics: what exactly is a physician assistant? Physician assistants (note: there is no apostrophe in the title) are asked this question often, because while the profession is growing and more patients are receiving care, it is often the first time this mid-level care has come directly from a PA. When someone asks me this question, my response usually goes something like this:

A PA is a healthcare provider who works with a doctor. A PA can perform many of the same functions that doctors can, with or without their physical supervision. For example, PAs can prescribe medications, perform procedures, perform physical exams, assist in surgeries, etc...

I then try to tailor the rest of my response to the setting, giving more clinical information if I am speaking with a patient. I certainly always try to answer the question in the most "real-life" way I can, because many people working outside of healthcare, who have not met a PA before, are unfamiliar with what we, as PAs, do. While some PA professionals shy away from saying that our work, "is somewhere between a physician and a nurse," I personally find that people usually grasp what you are trying to say if you describe it exactly that way.

For the technical definition of what a PA is, I will leave that up to professional organizations, such as the American Academy of Physician Assistants (the "AAPA"). According to the AAPA, the title "physician assistant" is defined as the following:

Physician assistants are health care professionals licensed (or in the case of those employed by the federal government they are credentialed), to practice medicine with physician supervision. As part of their comprehensive responsibilities, PAs conduct physical exams, diagnose and treat illnesses, order and interpret tests, counsel on preventive health care, assist in surgery, and write prescriptions. Within the physician-PA relationship, physician assistants exercise autonomy in medical decision making and provide a broad range of diagnostic and therapeutic services. A physician assistant's practice may also include education, research, and administrative services. PAs are trained in intensive education programs accredited by the Accreditation Review Commission on Education for the Physician Assistant ("ARC-PA"). Because of the close working relationship the PAs have with physicians, PAs are educated in the medical model designed to complement physician training. Upon graduation, physician assistants take a national certification examination developed by the National Commission on Certification of PAs in conjunction with the National Board of Medical Examiners. To maintain their national certification, PAs must log 100 hours of continuing medical education every two years and sit for a recertification every six years. Graduation from an accredited physician assistant program and passage of the national certifying exam are required for state licensure.[1]

That may be a little long-winded for your next cocktail party. However, be prepared for this question once you share your desire to attend PA school with your close friends or family. You may be the first PA they come into contact with, and you will want to portray your new profession in the most positive light possible—and part of that means having a ready answer for what you do—or will do. You could also let them know that, according to recent statistics from the Center for Disease Control and Prevention, of the nearly 1 billion patient office visits per year, patients were seen by a PA at about 36 million of those visits. Even if you do not decide to become a physician assistant in the future, it is likely that you or a loved one will be evaluated or treated by one in the future.

Key Characteristics of the Physician Assistant Role

The relationship between a PA and his or her supervising physician is unique in the healthcare setting. Most supervising physicians rely on their physician assistants to provide high quality care to their patients

---

[1] American Academy of Physician Assistants. Available at: http://www.aapa.org. Accessed December 6, 2011.

for them in those physicians' absence. Thus, physician assistants can become extensions of their supervising physicians. This does mean that the relationship between the PA and his or her supervising physician needs to be based on mutual trust and respect, and good communication.[2] Ultimately, while the physician is responsible for the care of the patient, the PA plays a large role in the way that care is provided.

Some PAs experience a great deal of autonomy within their work-setting. The amount of autonomy a PA has in his or her job will depend both upon the setting and the relationship with the supervising physician. Again, no matter what the level of autonomy, the physician must always be available for consultation with the PA. This consultation can occur in person or via some method of telecommunication (phone, e-mail, pagers, etc.). Some PAs work in clinics where their supervising physician is never in person, so these PAs act as the sole provider. However, because PAs are always subject to physician supervision, this type of work environment is only possible when the supervising physician has made arrangements to be available for contact at any time of day. PAs who work in this type of setting experience a great deal of autonomy and responsibility, but they must not forget the extent of their scope of practice.

Other PAs work directly with their supervising physician throughout the day. These PAs actually see patients together with their physician and participate in procedures together. As long as the PA is working within the scope of practice designated by his or her supervising physician, he or she is doing the job appropriately. Just remember the cardinal rule for PA practice: **the physician must be available for consult.**

---

[2] Hohman, J. Trust, Respect & Communication. PA Professional. April 2011.

How and Why was the PA Profession Created?

Although it may not seem important, it is worthwhile to understand how the PA profession began. (Additionally, it is possible that you will be asked this question during one your PA school interviews).

The demand for physician assistants grew out of a shortage of primary care physicians. In the 1960's, physicians realized that there was a need for additional healthcare providers who could treat patients in emergency situations and in underserved areas. Dr. Eugene Stead, a physician at Duke University, found a solution when he provided some ex-navy corpsmen with further training. The corpsmen were placed in a two-year experimental educational program, and when they were done, they were called physician assistants.[3]

That first program at Duke University officially began in 1965, and was limited to four students. Since then, the profession has expanded exponentially, and today there are 156 PA educational training programs, and more than 74,000 physician assistants in clinical practice.[4] It is likely that within the next few years this number will grow to include more than 100,000 practicing physician assistants! With the profession in its fourth decade, you will be joining the ranks of PAs during a period of fantastic growth.

Physician Assistant Scope of Practice

According to the AAPA, "the scope of the physician assistant's responsibilities corresponds to the supervising physicians' practice."[5] This simply means that, as a physician assistant, your scope of practice may be quite broad. In fact, that scope depends on what type of setting you work in, what the state medical boards allow, what hospital and/or clinics permit, and what your supervising physician allows.

---

[3] Physician Assistant History Center. Available at: http://www.pahx.org/index.htm. Accessed on July 5, 2011.
[4] American Academy of Physician Assistants. Available at: http://www.aapa.org. Accessed July 5, 2011.
[5] American Academy of Physician Assistants. Available at: http://www.aapa.org. Accessed August 1, 2011.

Although the duties vary from job to job, some of the typical PA responsibilities include:

- Completing patient histories and physical exams ("H & Ps")
- Acting as first assistant in the operating room
- Performing procedures as delineated by the supervising physician
- Providing assistance to the physician during procedures
- Evaluating, diagnosing, and treating new and existing patients' medical conditions
- Dictating patient care plans and treatment procedures
- Prescribing medications for patients (both inpatient and outpatient)
- Answering patient questions about procedures or treatment plans
- Ordering and interpreting laboratory values
- Ordering and interpreting radiology tests (x-rays, ultrasounds, CAT scans, and magnetic resonance imaging)
- Obtaining informed consent before procedures
- Documenting patient care plans and treatment procedures in each patient's chart

In addition to the work components listed above, there is a professional practice component to physician assistant practice. After completing an accredited program and passing the national certification exam, physician assistants are expected to embody certain "moral" and "professional" characteristics. Four PA organizations (the National Commission on Certification of Physician Assistants ("NCCPA"), the Accreditation Review Commission for Education of the Physician Assistant ("ARC-PA"), the Association of Physician Assistant Programs ("APAP"), and the AAPA) contributed to the creation of the "Physician Assistant Competencies" which were developed to ensure that PAs enhance quality and provide accountability in health care. As a PA, you will be expected to acquire and maintain the following six competencies:

- Medical knowledge
- Interpersonal and communication skills
- Patient care

- Professionalism
- Practice-based learning and improvement
- Systems-based practice

For a complete copy of these competencies, as well as more detailed information about them, please visit the National Commission on Certification of Physician Assistants' website at: http://www.nccpa.net.

How Does a Physician Assistant Make Money?

In order for PAs to be useful in the clinical setting, they must be cost-effective. Physician assistants can provide high quality patient care, and can reduce the cost of delivering that care. Over the years, various PA organizations have worked very hard to help create laws that allow physician assistants to be reimbursed by private insurance companies, Medicare, and Medicaid for the services they provide. This discussion may seem premature, but this topic may come up during PA school interviews, and it is a great subject to demonstrate the depth of your interest in becoming a PA. Keep in mind, information and policies do change frequently. And, there will be significant changes to the healthcare system and private insurance markets with the implementation of the Patient Protections and Affordable Care Act ("PPACA").[6]

Reimbursement from private insurance companies usually provides for the services provided by PAs, as long as those services are included as part of the physician's bill. The amount reimbursements cover will vary from insurance company to insurance company, and from state to state.

Physician assistants also receive reimbursement from Medicaid programs for services provided. As of now, all 50 states will provide reimbursement for amounts that are either the same as, or slightly lower than, the customary amounts paid to physicians. It is important to note

---

[6] Public Law 111 - 148 - Patient Protection and Affordable Care Act. Available at: http://www.gpo.gov/fdsys/pkg/PLAW-111publ148/content-detail.html Public Law 111 - 148 - Patient Protection and Affordable Care Act. Accessed July 6, 2011.

that, unlike other government programs, Medicaid is not mandated by federal laws that require reimbursement for services performed by PAs. This means each state can decide how services performed by physician assistants are billed and what the reimbursement rate is.[7]

Reimbursement for Medicare services is more complicated. In 1998, the Centers for Medicare and Medicaid Services ("CMS") revised its Medicare Carriers Manual reimbursement guidelines to include those services rendered by PAs. Medicare will reimburse for medical services provided by PAs in all settings at **85 percent** of the physician's customary fee, which is a significant improvement over past levels of reimbursement.[8] Bills to Medicare by physician assistants should include the PA's national provider identification number ("NPI"), signaling the patient was seen or treated by the PA and not the physician. Keep in mind, each state has its own specific laws—therefore, the reimbursement may be affected if services are not provided according to state law.

One exception to the above mentioned Medicare reimbursement rate is the idea of a "shared visit." In 2002, CMS issued new "Medicare Carriers Manual" instructions allowing PAs and physicians to bill at 100 percent of the physician's fee. This law requires that the physician and the PA work for the same employer or practice, and share visits made to patients the same day. This means that the physician must actually spend some "face-time" with the patient in order for the PA's service to be billed at 100 percent of the physician's fee. If the physician does not provide "face-time," the PA's patient visit may only be billed at the PA's fee of 85 percent. It is more lucrative for a physician to be on-site and seeing patients with the PA; however, for some physicians, billing at the PA's fee of 85 percent is just as profitable because it gives the physician time to participate in other aspects of patient care.

---

[7] American Academy of Physician Assistants. Available at: http://www.aapa.org/advocacy-and-practice-resources/reimbursement/medicaid. Accessed August 2, 2011.

[8] American Academy of Physician Assistants. Available at: http://www.aapa.org/advocacy-and-practice-resources/reimbursement/medicare/886-medicare-coverage-for-pas. Accessed on August 20, 2011.

There is another way services provided by a PA can be billed at 100 percent of the physician's fee: this provision of the law is called "incident-to," and applies to outpatient services that are provided in offices and clinics. There are four specific guidelines that must be followed in order to bill services at the physician's fee rate:

- The physician must be onsite when the PA is providing care;
- The physician must treat all new (first-visit) Medicare patients, as well as all established Medicare patients with a new medical condition;
- The PA must prescribe services that are within his or her scope of practice and are in accordance with the state's law; and
- The service rendered must be commonly performed in a physician's office.

Physician Assistants who work in the operating room as first assistants have slightly different reimbursement guidelines. Medicare provides reimbursement for a physician who first assists in the operating room at a rate of 16 percent of the primary surgeon's fee. When a PA first assists in the operating room, the billing percentage is less. The PA first assistant is reimbursed for 85 percent of the physician's first assistant rate of 16 percent, which means the PA first assistant will be reimbursed 13.6 percent of the primary surgeon's fee.[9]

As a PA, providing patient care is typically your most important duty. However, you must pay attention to billing as well. Reimbursement may be affected by improper billing, so PAs must learn to properly bill for their services—indeed, to bring revenue into a practice or hospital, a physician assistant must accurately bill for the services provided. Most PA programs will teach you basic concepts regarding how to bill, although, depending on the practice setting, the way you will bill for services will vary. Some private practice settings and hospitals have medical professionals (billing specialists and medical coders) who actually do the billing and coding for the physician and the physician

---

[9] American Academy of Physician Assistants. Available at: http://www.aapa.org/advocacy-and-practice-resources/reimbursement/medicare/892-first-assisting-at-surgery. Accessed August 22, 2011.

assistant which makes this part of a PA's job much easier.

Reimbursement can be extremely confusing. Even professional PAs sometimes find themselves confused about billing issues. For the most up-to-date information about physician assistant reimbursement, please visit the AAPA website at: www.aapa.org.

Opportunities for Physician Assistants

There has never been a better time to be a PA. And, if you pay attention to reports about "hot jobs," you will almost always see the PA profession at or near the top of the list. The United States Bureau of Labor Statistics ("BLS") projects that the number of PA jobs will increase by 39 percent between 2008 and 2018,[10] and in 2010, Money Magazine reported that being a PA was the second best job in America.[11]

Physician assistants are also in the national spotlight for what they do. In 2010, President Barack Obama recognized National Physician Assistant Week, marking the first time this celebration was acknowledged by a president. Physician assistant, Karen Bass, became the first PA member of the U.S. Congress, representing California's 33rd Congressional District, in 2011.[12] Physician Assistants even have their own radio show on ReachMD (XM160)!

In addition to having an in-demand job, you probably will not be bored. Physician assistant areas of practice are extremely varied, and PAs can work in any specialty they want to. PAs have opportunities to work in family practice, internal medicine, surgery, cardiothoracic surgery, dermatology, ophthalmology, obstetrics and gynecology…the opportunities are practically endless! Other countries have opened their doors to the concept of PAs as well, and physician assistants that were trained in America are currently working in both primary care and

---

[10] Bureau of Labor Statistics: United States Department of Labor. Available at: http://www.bls.gov/oco/ocos081.htm#outlook. Accessed June 22, 2011.
[11] CNN Money Magazine. *Best Jobs in America 2010*. Available at: http://money.cnn.com/magazines/moneymag/bestjobs/2010/full_list/. Accessed June 22, 2011.
[12] Kent, A. Mrs. Bass Goes to Washington. *PA Professional*, January 2011. Pages 21-22. Available at: http://paprofessional.cadmus.com//index.aspx?issue=01-jan-2011. Accessed August 1, 2011.

military settings in the United Kingdom, Canada, Australia, Saudi Arabia, Dubai, Egypt, and likely others.   The Canadian Medical Association now recognizes physician assistants as health professionals.   In addition to physician assistants practicing abroad, there are also training programs for PAs in Canada, Saudi Arabia, the United Kingdom, and Australia!

The work of a physician assistant is challenging, and may become even more demanding in the future.   In 2010, President Obama passed healthcare legislation that will help provide healthcare coverage to nearly 31 million uninsured Americans.   These 31 million Americans, who may not have been able to afford adequate healthcare in the past, will now have access to providers, including physician assistants. While this is wonderful news for patients, it also presents many challenges for physician assistants who might be see patients on those patients' first visits. It is likely that many of these patients have not received proper preventive care (such as immunizations or cancer screenings) in the past, and they may lack basic medical records and knowledge. This influx of new patients will likely increase the need for mid-level providers such as physician assistants and nurse practitioners who can help many of these patients in primary care settings.[13]

In sum, the opportunities for future physician assistants are endless. As the profession grows larger (and stronger because of its size), and the United States population continues to live longer, the job market for physician assistants is likely to be bright for years to come.

---

[13] Blumm, R. 31 Million New Patients are Coming. Are You Prepared? *Advance for PAs*. April 2011. Volume 2, Issue 4. Page 16.

Part II: Deciding to Become a Physician Assistant

Why Should I Become a Physician Assistant?

If you are reading this book, you (or someone you care about) are obviously thinking about applying to PA school. If attending PA school is a strong possibility for you, you should next ask yourself the following questions: "Do I really want to be a PA?" And, if so, "Why?" A long road follows these questions, and you must answer the first question with an honest "yes" if you are going to make it through the application process, through the education component, and then on to the challenging work you will face as a member of this profession.

Once you answer with a resounding "yes" and then determine what your motivations are, please take a moment to write them down. You will need to remind yourself of these reasons when you are stressed out or overwhelmed, and you may need to use these reasons to continue to inspire you. In fact, here are some of the initial reasons I wanted to be a PA. While they are only here for illustration, you might share at least some of my ideas—or these might inspire some of your own:

- **Opportunities to work collaboratively with physicians.** The relationship between physicians and physician assistants is unique. The idea of being able to work directly with a physician who respects me and the type of healthcare I could possibly provide was intriguing.
- **Opportunities to work in the operating room.** I loved the idea of giving expert assistance to a surgeon.
- **More opportunities for hands-on patient care.** As a dietitian, my role in the clinical setting was limited. I knew that if I became a PA, I would be able to do physical exams, participate in patient rounds, provide patient teaching, and prescribe medications.
- **Better pay.** Before working as a PA, I was only making about $30,000 a year, and I knew that with further schooling it would be possible to increase that substantially.

- **Opportunities to help people.**   Almost everyone who is drawn to healthcare wants to help people. PAs help people directly by seeing and treating patients, by providing education, and in countless other personal, hands-on ways.
- **Interests in medicine and surgery.** I love learning, and I am fascinated by science. I wanted classes and work experiences that would allow me to better understand the human body and how it functions.
- **Flexibility in scheduling.** Depending on the setting, physician assistants have the opportunity to work full-time, part-time, and/or per Diem. This was attractive to me because I wanted a profession that could provide family time, or time to pursue other academic or personal interests.
- **Opportunities to function like a physician, without years of medical school and residency training.** Saving both time and money were both important to me, but I did not want to give up the chance to practice hands-on healthcare.

What Does PA School Entail?

As I have said, being a physician assistant student is difficult. The course load is rigorous, and the expectations are high. Each student handles challenging education process differently. Some people have no problem balancing PA school with their outside lives; others find it overwhelming trying to keep up with the amount of material they are expected to retain.

The didactic, or classroom, portion of the PA program is typically the first year of the program and is usually the most difficult. Most programs require you to sit in class (and it is usually the same classroom!) anywhere from 8-12 hours per day, and then require you to study a few hours at night for a test the following morning. You generally have your weekends off, but will probably have to study on the weekends as well.

Luckily, after the didactic component, PA students begin the clinical portion of the program. Most students find the clinical portion much more enjoyable. While you will work long hours, including some overnight shifts, the clinical portion of most PA programs is much less mentally or "qualitatively" stressful because you have far fewer tests. However, the clinical portion is where students begin to feel the physical or "quantitative" demands of being a PA. Working in the operating room (the familiar "OR") for 12 hours, or participating in patient rounds on the floor that last 3-4 hours, will always be physically taxing on your body.

You can still have a life while you are a student, but you must prioritize your time wisely. Many students find the didactic portion of the program much more stressful simply because it is much more mentally onerous than the clinical portion of the program. What makes the didactic portion so difficult is that you are required to learn a great deal of complex medical information in a very short period of time.

Despite all of these warnings, PA school can be quite manageable. Most students who matriculate do end up completing the program, and every school wants all of its students to graduate. Realize at the outset what you are getting yourself into and, before it becomes overwhelming, find a way to manage the stress. Most students find an outlet.

Whether you choose exercise (or socializing, sleeping, watching television, journaling, etc.), if you are serious about going to PA school, you should carefully figure out your emotional profile, and determine how you can manage your stress beforehand. Make a personal plan now, and then begin your PA program with your plan in mind. This is one less thing to worry about when you are too exhausted to determine your next step.

And, contrary to everything I have already told you about PA school, please do not forget to have fun while you are attending school! This may be the only opportunity you have to live in a particular city, and will certainly be the last chance you will have to spend time with that particular group of students. Your fellow PA students are intelligent, dedicated people who share some of your ideals. Take advantage of this opportunity to make friends who may last a lifetime. Keep in mind that PA school is a temporary sacrifice—if your friends and family are aware of this they will likely respect your decision and support you throughout the program.

Aside from determining whether or not you really want to become a PA, there are other questions you must ask yourself before applying.

Do I Take Time off or Go Straight Through After College?

This is a difficult question to answer. Personally, I feel that those people who have taken time off after they have completed their undergraduate degree to actually gain some work experience in the healthcare field tend to have a better understanding of what working as a PA entails. If you have little or no healthcare experience, it is likely you will have little first-hand knowledge as to what a PA does and how much time and energy it takes to become one. However, if you have been working as a paramedic for two years while taking pre-requisites for PA school, you will probably have a much better idea of what a PA does and may demonstrate a greater appreciation for the opportunity to become one.

Most admissions committees prefer that you have healthcare experience. They like to see that you have worked "in the field" and that you have decided to become a PA because you have a solid understanding of the profession. If you demonstrate this type of experience, the committees will believe that you will make a better healthcare provider because you know how physicians, PAs, nurses, and other healthcare providers work—and work together.

Shadowing does not really provide a great deal of "hands on" healthcare experience; instead, shadowing is simply a way for you to get a glimpse of the profession. If you really want to be a PA, consider taking a year off after you complete your undergraduate degree to get substantial experience as a paramedic, nursing assistant, home health aid, or phlebotomist. Gaining actual work experience in the healthcare setting will benefit you as an applicant, and may round out your life as well.

On the other hand, if you have been planning to become a PA since high school and have been working in healthcare throughout your undergraduate education, go ahead and apply to PA school during your last year of school. Some students actually do better straight out of college, and you may be one of those lucky few. If you feel you have all the healthcare experience you want, and you have a solid understanding of the PA profession, you are a good candidate. Just be sure to make sure to highlight those parts of your application that clearly show your dedication.

Younger students who attend PA school directly after completing their undergraduate degrees sometimes appear immature in the work environment. While these students may do well in classroom and earn top grades, when thrown into clinical rotations they struggle. They may have (and demonstrate) little experience in the working world, and sometimes are oblivious to the fact that, as a student, they are at the bottom of the medical power structure.

Younger students tend to assume they are entitled to certain things—such as long lunch breaks, 3-day weekends, and unloading unappealing work (such as cleaning up body fluids) onto other healthcare workers. It is shocking to see intelligent people make such obvious professional mistakes. If you decide to continue your PA education directly after completing your undergraduate degree, keep in mind that working hard in the clinical setting is expected of you at all times. Make up for your lack of experience in the work environment by always demonstrating professionalism, a strong work ethic, and a positive attitude.

How Much does Physician Assistant School really Cost?

Simply put, school costs money. And, unfortunately, PA school costs **a lot** of money. For comparison's sake, and to give you your first sticker shock, I have listed the tuition numbers from several schools. Please note that this is only tuition; many schools tack on additional fees as well. Also, because these rates change frequently, I urge you to confirm any tuition rates with any and all schools you are specifically applying to.

Tuition costs at various PA programs for program duration (often about 2 years) as of July 2011:

- University of Alabama: $39,543 (in-state), $92,722 (out-of-state)[14]
- Arizona School of Health Sciences: $62,866[15]
- Loma Linda University: $78,120[16]
- Duke University: $61,733[17]
- Weill Medical College of Cornell University: $76,731[18]
- Barry University: $71,000[19]
- Central Michigan University: $60,172 (in-state), $94,892 (out-of-state)[20]
- Midwestern University: $81,005[21]
- Rosalind Franklin University: $53,528[22]
- University of Iowa: $38,370 (in-state), $79,914 (out-of-state)[23]
- Miami Dade Community College: $15,116 (in-state), $67,459 (out-of-state)[24]
- University of California – Davis: $30,381 (in-state), $53,403 (out-of-state)[25]

---

[14] University of Alabama Physician Assistant Program. Available at: http://www.uab.edu/shp/admissions-tuition/tuition/tuition-fees. Accessed on August 1, 2011.
[15] Arizona School of Health Sciences Physician Assistant Program. Available at: http://www.atsu.edu/ashs/programs/physician_assistant/tuition_expenses.htm. Accessed on August 1, 2011.
[16] Loma Linda University Physician Assistant Program. Available at: http://www.llu.edu/allied-health/sahp/admissions/tuition.page. Accessed on August 1, 2011.
[17] Duke University Physician Assistant Program. Available at: http://paprogram.mc.duke.edu/Admissions/Tuition. Accessed on August 1, 2011.
[18] Weill Medical College of Cornell University Physician Assistant Program. Available at: http://weill.cornell.edu/education/programs/handbook.html. Accessed on August 1, 2011.
[19] Barry University Physician Assistant Program. Available at: (http://www.barry.edu/pa/FinancialAid/programFees.htm. Accessed on August 1, 2011.
[20] Central Michigan University Physician Assistant Program. Available at: (http://www.cmich.edu/chp/x894.xml. Accessed on August 1, 2011.
[21] Midwestern University Physician Assistant Program. Available at: (http://www.midwestern.edu/Programs_and_Admission/AZ_Physician_Assistant_Studies.html#Estimated%20Cost%20of%20Attendance. Accessed on August 1, 2011.
[22] Rosalind Franklin University Physician Assistant Program. Available at: http://www.rosalindfranklin.edu/dnn/CHP/PA/MS/Tuition/tabid/1587/Default.aspx. Accessed on August 1, 2011.
[23] University of Iowa Physician Assistant Program. Available at: http://paprogram.medicine.uiowa.edu/Site/programinfo.html. Accessed on August 1, 2011.
[24] Miami Dade Community College Physician Assistant Program. Available at: http://www.mdc.edu/main/bashspa/tuition.asp. Accessed on August 1, 2011.
[25] University of California – Davis Physician Assistant Program. Available at: http://www.ucdmc.ucdavis.edu/medschool/financialaid/pdfs/1011-coa-fnppa.pdf. Accessed on August 1, 2011.

- Anne Arundel Community College: $19,226 (in-state), $40,537 (out-of-state)[26]
- Philadelphia University: $69,960[27]

If you are more curious and wish to compare further, you can find the estimated tuition costs for all 156 PA schools in this book's index.

These are estimates provided from the schools' websites. Remember, in addition to tuition costs, you should add an additional $20,000-$30,000 for room and board, transportation and personal expenses during the program. You will probably also need to add another $3,000-$4,000 for medical equipment, technology fees, books, and certification or licensing fees.

The cost to attend PA school (depending on where you go) will total around $50,000-$160,000. Now, if you go to an in-state program and live at home with your parents or family, your costs will be substantially lower—but even then, there are no guarantees. And, either way, this is a significant investment of both time and money.

Making the Commitment to Become a Physician Assistant

If you are reading this book, you have already demonstrated some interest in the profession. However, reading a book is one thing; the arduous process of application, attendance, paying down student loan debt, and practice is a long road. I urge you to please spend some quiet moments carefully testing your commitment to becoming a PA before you even apply. Attending PA school is extremely difficult and requires a significant investment of time and money. You must be completely dedicated to the program and the profession in order to

[26] Anne Aurndel Community College Physician Assistant Program. Available online at: http://www.aacc.edu/tuitionfees/. Accessed on August 1, 2011.
[27] Philadelphia University Physician Assistant Program. Available online at: http://www.philau.edu/paprogram/pacost.htm. Accessed on August 1, 2011.

successfully become a PA. This career is not for everyone; rather, this career is for people who are willing to dedicate two (or more) long years of their lives to learning all they possibly can about medicine and surgery. Remember, PAs do not need to complete a residency program like physicians. PAs get their substantive training solely during their academic program, so you must learn all you can in those two years before you are practicing.

As a PA student, you will sacrifice a great deal of your free time so that you can study and learn the necessary information to practice medicine competently—even information not presented in class. You must be prepared to take on this challenge willingly. Many practicing PAs view their training as a condensed form of medical school. However, medical school lasts four years (without clinical residencies), and PA school (including its clinical portion) are little more than two compressed years of education.

Unlike medical school, PA school typically provides students with only the necessary science and health information that students will need in order to practice medicine or surgery effectively. This means that you will likely need to fill in any gaps in your knowledge base on your own. For example, you may not have coursework that is dedicated to microbiology in PA school, which means you may need to review this information on your own in order to be successful in some of the courses.

As an educator, I have seen students fail out of PA programs (or struggle through them) because they were not devoting the necessary time to studying. While I believe many of these students were capable of succeeding in the program had they dedicated themselves appropriately, practically speaking, not everyone is cut out for the intensity of studying that is required during the educational process.

You must realistically assess the cost of attending PA school. As mentioned before, tuition costs keep rising, and upon graduation most PA school graduates have some form of student loan debt. Many PA programs do not allow students to work during the programs (for good reason). Realize that you will likely have no income during the period of time you are a PA student, because there is no free time for part-time work. If you are not willing to take on these costs, you may not be able to become a PA. Another consideration is this: if you begin a PA program, you do not want to fail or "wash out." If this happens, you will end up in the worst possible situation: you will not have the degree you paid money towards, and you will be stuck paying back loans regardless of your personal circumstances.

It is important to have a good support system in place before you begin PA school, because it is likely that you will need to rely on others at times during your education. If you have a family, make sure they support your decision to attend PA school. Your immediate family must understand that you will be in class almost all day long, and that you will be required to study nearly every night. If you have children, you need to make sure you are willing to miss out on some parts of their lives during your education. You will also need to make sure you have the appropriate child care in place to help assist you during the time you are in school. Your family should understand that you may be working night-shifts during your clinical rotations. They must remember that you will not be able to contribute income during the time you are in PA school.

If you decide to attend, make sure your family and friends (especially your family) are well aware of the sacrifices everyone will have to make. I have seen many students struggle emotionally due to the stress they are under during PA school. It was quite common for students to cry in my office as they expressed some of the difficulties they were experiencing emotionally, due to school issues, home issues, or some combination of the two.

Life will continue happening while you are in school, and sometimes there are issues out of your control that will affect your emotional well-being. For example, a family member may become sick or your spouse may lose his or her job while you are in school. These are all real possibilities that you must be prepared to deal with. Again, it is paramount that you have a solid support system in place before you begin school, as it is likely that you will need a hug here and there, and possibly a shoulder to cry on occasionally. If you are the one supplying the hugs and the shoulders exclusively, your PA school path will be much more difficult, and the odds against your success will mount.

Understanding the Differences between Mid-Level Providers and Physicians

The question of "who do I want to be" is critical for anyone who wants to become a health care provider, especially someone facing years of specialized education and training. You do not want to push yourself through the academic rigors of becoming a PA, and then realize you really wanted to be a medical doctor ("MD"), doctor of osteopathic medicine ("DO"), nurse practitioner ("NP"), or another type of healthcare professional.

To help make sure you understand the role each of these professions plays in the healthcare model, as well as the educational requirements to satisfy the requirements to be one, I will take you through the current (as of 2011) basic requirements to become a PA, MD, DO, or NP, as well as some of their basic functions in healthcare below. This will also help you to be conversant about common clinical professions if you are asked about them during your PA school interviews.

Physician Assistant

To become a PA, you must successfully complete the educational requirements of one of the accredited PA programs in the United States. PA Programs are typically 24-27 months in length, and combine both a didactic component and a clinical component. PAs are required to take and pass a certifying exam as well as obtain state licensure before they can practice. PAs are considered mid-level providers, and, under the guidance of a supervising physician, they are licensed to provide medical care autonomously in many different settings. Currently, the terminal degree for physician assistants is a Masters degree. However, there is one clinical doctoral program that already practicing physician assistants in the military may enroll in.[28,29]

---

[28] Raines, F. The Doctor of Nursing Practice: A Report on Progress. American Association of Colleges of Nursing. Available online at: http://www.aacn.nche.edu/DNP/pdf/DNPForum3-10.pdf. Accessed on August 22, 2011.
[29] American Association of Colleges of Nursing Program List. Available online at: http://www.aacn.nche.edu/DNP/DNPProgramList.htm. Accessed on August 22, 2011.

Nurse Practitioner

To become a nurse practitioner, you must first complete a registered nurse training program, followed by successful completion of the educational requirements at one of the accredited NP programs in the United States. Several NP programs are about 2 years in length and provide graduates with a master's degree. However, this is slowly changing as the American Association of Colleges of Nursing ("AACN") has recommended that all nurse practitioner programs provide graduates with a doctoral degree for entry-level practice beginning in 2015.[28]

Nurse practitioners are advanced practice nurses and are required to take (and pass) a certifying exam and obtain state licensure before they can practice. NPs are considered mid-level providers, and they do not universally require physician supervision. NPs receive specialized training in one specific area of practice, however, they are able to work in sub-specialty areas if they desire to. PAs and NPs are both mid-level providers. However, there are some differences between the two professions: NPs are trained in one area of practice (for example, family health or acute care), but do not universally require physician supervision.

In contrast, PAs are not trained in one specific are of practice and can work in any type of healthcare setting (for example, surgery or family practice), but PAs *do* require physician supervision. MDs or DOs are not mid-level providers and they do not require supervision by other physicians. They take on extensive medical or surgical training so they can appropriately treat their patients, with or without the help of other physicians or mid-level providers.

Physician

To become a MD or a DO, you must successfully complete an undergraduate degree, as well as the educational requirements of an accredited medical school program. Medical school consists of approximately 4 years of graduate level education, and combines both didactic and clinical components. After graduating from medical school, you must apply to a residency program that provides approximately 3-7 years of additional training under the supervision of senior physician educators. Following the completion of a residency, you may (or may not) decide to complete a fellowship lasting approximately 1-3 years if you want specialized training. Doctors are required to take a series of certification examinations throughout medical school, residency, and at the completion of their training. Doctors must also obtain a license to practice medicine in the state in which they work.

Doctors are extensively trained because they are ultimately responsible for the treatment and management of their patients. In contrast to PAs, if a physician wanted to switch to another "field," he or she would have to complete an additional residency. Physicians are independent practitioners and can practice completely on their own.

If you are interested in learning even more about these professions and their differences, I encourage you to review each websites devoted to each profession. The following websites are filled with interesting content about how each profession began, the current training requirements, current issues facing each profession, and much more:

- American Academy of Physician Assistants:
  http://www.aapa.org
- American Academy of Nurse Practitioners:
  http://www.aanp.org
- American Medical Association: http://www.ama-assn.org
- American Association of Colleges of Osteopathic Medicine:
  http://www.aacom.org

Mid-Level Providers

The term "mid-level provider" is an umbrella title that refers to any non-physician healthcare practitioner. As a PA, you must be familiar with this term and its nuances because it typically includes both physician assistants and nurse practitioners. Many physician assistants and nurse practitioners do not like this title, as they believe it suggests that there are professions that are "higher" and "lower" than PAs and NPs. In fact, some of the professional NP and PA organizations have urged lawmakers to stop using this term in legislation.[30] Although the original design for the roles of NPs and PAs was quite different, for both economic and healthcare access reasons, the difference between these clinicians has decreased and the scopes of practice have sometimes blended. To help you get a better understanding of the two professions, I want to review some of the similarities and differences between the two:

Similarities:

- Both PAs and NPs are considered mid-level providers
- Both PAs and NPs can prescribe medications
- Both PAs and NPs can work with supervising physicians
- Both PAs and NPs as a profession have been practicing since the 1960's
- Both PAs and NPs must pass a certification exam in order to practice
- Both PAs and NPs must have licenses to practice, depending on state laws
- Both PAs and NPs are eligible for certification as Medicaid and Medicare providers

Differences:

- PAs are trained after the "medical model" in the same manner as physicians. PA training is disease centered, with its emphasis on the biological/pathological and psychological/social aspects of health, assessment, diagnosis and treatment. Clinical training for PAs often exceeds 2,000 hours
- NPs are trained in the "nursing model" which is specific to nurses, biopsychosocial centered, with emphases on health promotion, wellness, and prevention. Clinical training hours for

---

[30] Mittman, D. Let's End the Dreaded Term Mid-Level. Clinician1. Available at: http://clinician1.com//posts/article/lets_end_the_dreaded_term_midlevel. Accessed on June 28, 2011.

NPs range from approximately 500-700 hours. (Keep in mind, nurse practitioners have clinical training hours as registered nurses that are not included in this hourly total)

- PAs are dependent practitioners and are required to have a supervising physician
- NPs are independent practitioners and can practice without supervision (depending on the state)
- PAs have different backgrounds before becoming PAs (such as paramedics, nurses, radiology techs, medical assistants, dietitians, phlebotomists, etc.)
- NPs must first be registered nurses ("RNs") before becoming NPs
- PAs can provide services in any specialty, under guidelines defined by a supervising physician, state, or hospital
- NPs are specialized in one type of clinical practice, such as Family Medicine, Neonatology, etc. (This does not, however, mean they cannot practice in a sub-specialty)

As you can see, there are good reasons why people sometimes confuse the two professions. In certain settings, we both provide the same services and work alongside one another. However, as a future PA it is important that you understand the differences between the two professions, and make sure you are practicing according to the guidelines appropriate for a PA.

It is important to understand that nurse practitioners and physician assistants often function in collaborative relationships. These relationships are based on both professions acknowledging our shared values and commitment to providing high quality service, and an understanding that cooperation is necessary to provide proper care. This relationship is often unique, based on the scope of practice for a specific job (which may vary from state to state), and practice regulations that can influence the level and degree of collaboration within a practice site. One thing is clear: a collaborative relationship in the workplace dramatically increases the standard of care and quality of outcomes.[31]

Final Thoughts on Deciding Whether or Not the PA Profession is Right for You

If you have followed the steps of the book thus far, you have done a fair bit of work to consider why the profession may be the best career option for you. However, some people want to be a PA for the wrong reasons—and, you might be one of those people. This section could help you recognize that before you apply and become a PA student— and before you regret the decision.

There are a number of reasons why I would discourage some people from becoming a PA. You might be applying to PA school as your "back-up" plan for medical school. Some applicants apply to PA school because they were not accepted to medical school, or because they want a safety plan in case they do not get accepted to medical school.

If you are considering applying to PA school "just in case" plan A does not work out, please save your application money. Our profession needs people who truly want to be PAs and not doctors. And, why would you want to spend all that money to become a PA, only to realize five years down the road that you still want to go to medical school? If you want to be a doctor, apply to medical school. If you truly wish to go, there are many viable options.

You should reconsider becoming a PA if you do not like caring for sick individuals. Physician assistants, like many other healthcare workers, treat patients with a variety of medical conditions. Sometimes the duties of a PA require true compassion. It is routine for physician assistants to perform rectal examinations, clean out infected wounds,

---

[31] Lavoie-Vaughan, N. Collaborative practice: Understanding is the key. Available online at: http://www.advanceweb.com/NPPA. Advance for NPs & PAs. June 2011. **Volume 2, Issue 6:** Page 17. Accessed on August 22, 2011.

suction secretions from tracheostomies, and care for confused or combative patients. Please consider this carefully. If you are not comfortable helping someone who may vomit all over you mid-examination, than this may not be the profession for you.

If you cannot make the commitment to two or three years of dedicated study, please avoid PA school. Almost every PA program has one or two students who do not make it from entry through graduation, and this ends up being unfortunate for everyone involved. I realize that life sometimes throws unexpected obstacles at us, but if you decide to attend a program, you must be whole-heartedly committed. Dropping out of a PA program halfway through costs you a lot of time and a lot of money, and it also keeps other deserving students from having the opportunity to enter a program. So, if you are commitment-phobic, please consider a different career path.

You should reconsider becoming a PA if you are in the profession **solely** for money or for prestige. Yes, PAs make a good living, but they work very hard. PAs also invest a lot of money into their education, which means many PAs carry significant student loan debt.

As far as prestige goes, physician assistants have an important place in the medical setting. However, PAs will never have the prestige that physicians have (nor the tremendous amount of responsibility), and from my experience, most PAs do not actively seek prestige. Those that do are the distinct minority and, stick out like a sore thumb. Most PAs I have studied with or practiced with simply want to provide quality healthcare to their patients.

Finally, you should reconsider becoming a PA if you simply cannot think of anything else to do with your life. This is not the ideal postpone-your-career path or default option, and no one views PA school as the "go to law school post-BA" solution for science majors. Becoming a PA takes complete dedication to the program you are attending, and practicing as a PA requires that same dedication to our profession as a whole.

As an added thought, for each of the reasons above, it will be extremely difficult to do well as a student in a rigorous PA program if you really do not begin with the drive or desire to be a part of the profession. Think carefully, think often, and think a final time before you drop your application—or your deposit check—in the mail.

Researching the Competition: Who is the "Average" PA Student?

Each year, the AAPA conducts a survey to collect census information from the PA profession. (And, if and when you become a PA, I strongly urge you to participate in this survey as it is useful to the entire profession). This census information allows us to view various statistical data about the profession, including information about PA students. If you would like to access this information, it is listed publicly on the AAPA website. It is important to note that this information changes from year to year, so it is likely that some of the information is already a bit outdated. However, it still demonstrates where the PA profession is trending.

The "Average" Student

According to the AAPA's most recent census information, here is what you need to know about the "average" PA student before you apply:[32]

- The average PA student is 25.2 years old
- 71% of PA students are female
- 8% of PA students have military experience
- 28% of PA students are married
- 79% of PA students are white/Caucasian
- 50% of PA students have a bachelor's degree in biology
- 79% of PA students had worked in healthcare prior to applying (either part-time or full-time)
- 27% of PA students had less than one year of healthcare work experience prior to applying

---

[32]American Academy of Physician Assistants. Available at: http://www.aapa.org. Accessed June 28, 2011.

- 17% of PA students were Emergency Medical Technicians before PA school
- 18% of PA students were medical assistants before PA school
- 40% of PA students only applied to one PA school
- 31% of PA students applied to more than 4 schools
- 83% of PA students were accepted to one PA program on their first application
- The mean accepted PA students' undergraduate GPA is a 3.5
- The mean amount of expected student loan debt incurred during PA school is $55,321
- 44% of PA students plan to work in family practice/internal medicine
- 37% of PA students plan to work in emergency medicine
- 33% of PA students plan to work in surgical specialties

If you are an applicant with an undergraduate degree in biology and a GPA of 3.5, with some healthcare experience, you are very likely to be accepted to PA school (and will blend in well). However, if you are a 37 year-old engineer trying to apply to PA school, does that mean you will not be accepted? Of course not. These statistics are included to demonstrate who the average PA student is so you can make an informed decision. Remember, not all PA students fall into the "average" category. Personally, I have no desire to be average—and I imagine that you feel the same.

Physician Assistant School Acceptance Criteria

Every school has its own rating system for their selection or rejection of applicants. Fortunately, some of this information is quite standard even among different programs, and you can use the standard criteria to best position yourself for success.

Most schools have a "points" system which they use to rank their applicants, and this points system is often calculated from the information received from the Central Application Service for

Physician Assistants ("CASPA").[33] CASPA is the online application program that many programs require applicants to use in order to apply to PA school. (We will talk more about using the CASPA when we discuss the application process).   After a school receives your information from the CASPA, they typically give you a certain number of points based on the initial information they receive about you.

Making a Strong First Impression

Like most graduate programs, and more so as PA school becomes more popular, PA schools receive many more applications than they have available space for; thus they must "weed" out the more unqualified students early on before spending more time on more promising candidates. Your first goal as an applicant is to avoid being "weeded," and the CASPA application you submit is your first opportunity. The CASPA speaks on your behalf, and makes a strong first impression. This is the first glimpse of you that any school will get, so carefully review everything before you submit it.

Most schools review your initial application and give you points based on:

- Overall grade point average ("GPA")
- Natural science GPA
- Non-science GPA
- GRE score
- Any graduate credits or degrees you have earned. (These may give you additional credits depending on the school)
- Healthcare experience
- Letters of Recommendation

---

[33] Centralized Application System for Physician Assistants. Available online at: https://portal.caspaonline.org. Accessed August 22, 2011.

Some schools may add or subtract additional points based on:

- Quality of education: Did you attend a community college, an Ivy League-type of school, or somewhere in between?
- Quality of healthcare experience: Did you obtain direct patient care (hands-on) experience, or indirect patient care?
- Length of healthcare experience: Did you work as a nursing assistant for two years, or did you shadow a PA for only two days?
- Grade trends: Did you have a low GPA semester early on? If so, did your grades consistently improve following that point?
- Age of academic experience: Did you last complete a science course more than 5-10 years ago?
- Desire to work in a specific setting: Did you apply to a school that is dedicated to providing healthcare in medically underserved areas? If so, did you support your desire to do that type of work on your application?
- The schools will also review your personal statement and will award points based on the quality of the statement. This makes it important to write a great personal statement, which is something we will talk about further in the book. Sometimes the program will also review your letters of recommendation before moving you onto the next round of the application process; however, many times PA faculty do not review these letters unless and until you have received an interview from the school.
- Based on the above information, the school will calculate your total points, and if you meet the school's minimum criteria, you may be granted a secondary or supplemental application, or a personal interview. If you receive either of these, you should be ecstatic! It means that you have met the minimum requirements for admission, you have avoided being "weeded" out, and that you will now have the opportunity to further explain why you want to attend PA school—and why you will someday make a wonderful, competent PA.

Characteristics of Strong Applicants

Successful applicants are able to demonstrate to admissions officers that they would be an asset to the PA program to which they are applying, and there are several things you can do as an applicant to increase your chances of gaining admission into a physician assistant educational program.

Grade Point Average

First and foremost, focus on your grades. The initial item each school reviews is your GPA, and this typically carries the most weight in the initial points calculation process. If you only have a 2.5 GPA, getting into PA school is going to be very difficult. You must improve your GPA if you want to be competitive. I know the thought of taking additional classes simply to improve your GPA may be costly and tedious, but if you are committed to being a PA, you may need to do just that. This factor may also focus your decision to even apply.

If you have a lower GPA, you should consider taking additional classes (I recommend science) or repeat courses you did poorly in. If you are simply trying to add a few classes to boost your GPA, you may want to consider taking your additional classes at a community college—it is less expensive and sometimes less intense. However, some programs frown upon community college courses, so you must take this into consideration as well.

It is common for students to retake science courses, so do not beat yourself up if you did poorly in a class or two and realize that you need to take the course again. Let me share a secret with you: I am imperfect. In fact, the first time I took organic chemistry in college, I received a failing grade. By re-enrolling in the course, I actually began to understand the material and found it interesting, rather than just confusing. Additionally, I was motivated to do well in the class to prove to myself and my professors that I was capable of succeeding. (I will also admit that paying for a course a second time is another great motivating force).

PA educators realize that students are human too. They understand that sometimes you have extenuating circumstances that impact your ability to succeed in a course (or, in some cases, an entire semester of school). If you find yourself in a situation where you are not performing as well as you had hoped, meet with the professor of the course as soon as possible so that you can discuss ways to improve your grade. And, if you realize that you bit off more than you can chew, try to drop the course or withdraw before you actually receive a failing grade.

Graduate Record Examination

In addition to having a good GPA, you will probably need to do well on the Graduate Record Examination ("GRE"). (Be sure to check whether or not your school requires you to take the GRE because not all schools do). To find out more information about the GRE, you may visit the official GRE website at: http://www.ets.org/gre.

Whether you are taking the GRE for the first time, or are retaking it, I recommend that you purchase a study aid. (I wish someone had emphasized the importance of this to me before I took the exam the first time!). Although books and study programs can be costly, doing well on the exam is important as you will need to prove that you are capable of succeeding on a standardized exam. PA schools want to have students who can successfully pass the Physician Assistant National Certification Exam ("PANCE") on their first attempt. By doing well on the GRE, you are demonstrating that you will likely do well on the PANCE after you graduate.

Every student uses different methods to study. After years of taking computerized examinations, I have found that the best way for me to learn is by doing practice exams. By completing a practice exam, you are able to get a general idea of how you might score on an actual examination. This information is incredibly helpful, as it can help you identify areas of weakness—thus, giving you some insight as to what you need to focus on before actually taking the exam.

The study-aid agencies have books you may use to study for the GRE, as well as online and in-person programs you can purchase. To get you started, here are the most well-known study guides for the GRE:

- Kaplan (http://www.kaptest.com)
- Princeton Review (http://www.princetonreview.com)

There are plenty of other study books or programs available. If money is an issue, you can purchase used books online at reduced prices. Additionally, it is likely that your local library has plenty of books available for you to borrow. Some universities have their own resources and study groups available for students to use—you may even discover that your university offers tutoring programs specific for the GRE. Whatever method you decide to use, make sure you do *something* to prepare.

The scoring system for the GRE is a bit complicated, as it has three sections that are each scored differently. The scoring system has recently been revised (and it may change again by the time you are reading this), so forgive me if this information is not accurate. Presently, the scoring ranges for the exam are between 130-170 on the Verbal section,   130-170 on the Quantitative section, and a score of 0-6 on the Analytical writing section. To be competitive, you should try to achieve a score in the 70th percentile in each section. Many schools do not have a minimum score for acceptance into their programs, but I would advise you to check with each school to find out what your prospective schools require. Some PA program websites will list the "average" scores from the previous group of admitted students. This can be particularly useful as a guide for your application.

I have noticed there are trends in GRE scores among PA students. Students who are stronger in the sciences tend to score higher on the Analytical and Quantitative sections of the GRE than they do on the Verbal sections. If you notice your score demonstrates this paradigm, do your best to decide whether or not having a deficiency in one area is worth retaking the exam. If you do need to retake the exam, work on strengthening your scores in the weakest areas by using a GRE prep book or flashcards.

Being a PA means you will have to take multiple computerized examinations for competency in the future, so you cannot shy away from computerized exams. Do your best to prepare for the exam appropriately, and if this is your first computer test, take advantage of the professional computerized exam experience.

Clinical Experience

Before you apply to PA school, you *must* get some clinical experience! There is no excuse for not having any exposure to healthcare before you apply. I do realize that some people have no idea where to start. If you have a degree in English and want to be a PA, how do you get experience working in a hospital or clinic? It is much easier than you think.

Most schools prefer that applicants have "hands-on" patient care experience. This means exactly what it sounds like: you are working in a setting that allows you to touch the patients. An example might be a nurse, or a phlebotomist. Realistically, it is quite easy to get this type of health experience—it just takes a little bit of time, training, and may take some money.

The easiest thing you can do is to become a nursing or medical assistant. To do this, you will be required to complete a course (usually anywhere from two weeks to six months) in order to work as a certified nursing assistant ("CAN"), a personal care assistant ("PCA"), or a medical assistant ("MA"). The classes are worth it because you will learn skills that will be useful in your future career as a PA, and when you do get a job as a nursing assistant, you will be getting paid to hone your skills.

Another option for getting hands-on experience is becoming an emergency medical technician ("EMT") or a paramedic. Again, you must complete a course in order to do this, and courses range anywhere from six months in length to two years. The EMTs and paramedics I matriculated with were extremely knowledgeable about the role of the PA and about patient care in general. They also had some of the highest grades in PA school, perhaps because of their experience. If you have the time and the money, I highly recommend this type of training.

If you are looking for a quick way to get some experience, take a phlebotomy course. Some phlebotomy courses can be taken in only one weekend. After you have received your certification, you can apply for a job in a hospital and get some experience drawing blood. Any of these paths to direct patient care will benefit you in your journey to becoming a PA.

The latest "craze" for pre-PA and pre-medical students is to work as a medical scribe. A medical scribe is a person who enters the patient room with physician and types up the patient's medical information during the interview. This service makes it easier for the physician to format his or her medical records as they can easily pull items from the draft the medical scribe has created. It can also be helpful for physicians as they see multiple patients each day and may not remember all of the details about each encounter.

Working as a medical scribe is considered valuable experience for pre-PA students as the student has to learn a variety of important clinical skills. Some of these skills you may learn include: how to work in a fast-pace medical environment, how to use medical terminology and medical abbreviations appropriately, how to conduct a patient interview, and how to work with demanding (and not always nice) healthcare providers.

Generally, immersing yourself in the mindset of a physician can give you a greater understanding of the world of healthcare in the United States. For more information about working as a scribe, do an online search. You will find many companies provide training to eager undergraduate students who are willing to commit to working for them for a year or two.

As you can see, these jobs require some training. This means that you will need to think about obtaining this training early, and you will need to be proactive. If you are reading this as a freshman or sophomore in college, take these courses during the summer or during a semester of school when your course load is a bit lighter (if such a semester exists).

If you can work at a local hospital or in a physician's office while you are still in school, this will make obtaining these patient contact hours much easier. Planning is key for making this happen. Look to local community colleges or hospitals for training programs and schedules, and enroll early—these programs fill up quickly.

I was personally quite lucky in that I studied dietetics in undergrad, so I was able to get substantive healthcare experience as part of my program. If you are in an undergraduate program that allows you to participate in an internship in a healthcare setting, take advantage of this. Discuss your future goals with your adviser and ask for assistance with obtaining the most useful type of patient care experience available.

If, for some reason, you do not have sufficient time or are unable to find a job that will allow you to get "hands-on" experience, you should still try to get non-direct patient care experience. You can do this by signing up to be a hospital volunteer, by shadowing a PA or doctor, or by working in a clinic. Contact local physicians' offices to see if there are opportunities to observe or work (in some capacity) in those offices.

Also, some people in PA school have healthcare experience from work as health educators in different types of settings. There are even some former drug-reps who attend PA school. So, because the opportunities to get "healthcare" experience are as limitless as your creativity, you should be able to find something that fits into your schedule and that will benefit you as you attempt to apply to and succeed in PA school.

If you are still in high school, or are just beginning your college career, that is excellent—insofar as you have plenty of time to plan ahead. I would encourage you to start obtaining useful training opportunities as early as possible. Having a variety of experiences will enable you to stand out, and make you more likely to succeed in the profession because you will have a better understanding of the role of the physician assistant.

If you are able to start early, and to maximize your standing as a highly competitive applicant, you should consider all of the following potential experiences, and determine which sound the most appealing:

- Physician assistant shadowing over several years (and in several different settings)
- Physician shadowing (because it is important to understand the differences between the professions)
- Working as a medical scribe throughout college to learn more about patient care
- Taking an emergency medical technician course or certified nursing assistant course, (then passing the exam), and subsequently working in this field
- Taking a phlebotomy course—or trying to work in an environment where you can obtain these skills
- Taking first aid and/or cardiopulmonary resuscitation courses
- Volunteering in local hospitals or nursing homes
- Joining the Pre-PA club at your university to learn of other unique opportunities

Do not just *do* these tasks—concurrently *document* them as well. Documenting all of these experiences in your application will demonstrate your commitment to the profession, your ability to plan accordingly, your ability to manage your time appropriately, and your desire to learn all you can about working in the healthcare field.

Documenting will also show that you are organized, and you will not have to hunt down specific dates or the names of physicians, hospitals, or trainers when you start filling out your application. You will definitely stand out if you have multiple certifications and health-care related experiences. You will also have a lot of material to draw from in your personal narrative and during your interview.

All is not lost if you do not begin obtaining these experiences until your senior year of college. However, if you hope to matriculate into a PA program shortly after graduation, you will have a much more difficult time finding a way to fit things in. You will have to find opportunities that will give you the most "bang for your buck" and will allow you to maximize your logged, patient-care hours. It should be clear that it is much easier to schedule things over the course of several months and years, but the options discussed above should still be considered one after another.

Shadowing Experience

I mentioned shadowing in the previous paragraph. Regardless of your background, many PA schools express a preference that you have some shadowing experience before you apply. Personally, I believe this is an absolute necessity. Shadowing a PA will help confirm your understanding of the PA profession, and highlight the difference between a PA and a physician. If you know any PAs, ask them if they would let you shadow them. Sometimes PAs will let you shadow them for months; other times they may only allow you to come in and follow them for a few hours. It depends on the PA, and it depends on the setting. And do not take a negative response personally—because of the Health Insurance Portability and Accountability Act ("HIPAA") laws, some hospitals and clinics may not allow students to shadow because it "may affect patient confidentiality."

While I respect personal privacy and the law protecting it, it certainly makes getting shadowing experience more difficult. If you find a PA who says you cannot shadow them because HIPAA laws do not allow students in their organization, do not give up. You should contact other PAs or doctors to find out if they can help you find someone to shadow. You should also contact a local PA or Medical school program and ask if they know anyone who may be able to help you. And, if you still cannot find anyone, you should contact some of the professional organizations and ask them for help (for example, your state PA organization, the AAPA, AASPA, AFPPA, etc.).

There is an online tool that may aid you in finding a PA to shadow. A physician assistant in California created the PA Shadow Online website to help connect practicing physician assistants with students looking to gain shadowing experience. The website is definitely worth exploring if you are hoping to obtain PA shadowing experience. You can view the website at: http://www.pashadowonline.com.

Once you have found someone to shadow, you should take advantage of that opportunity to learn first-hand what a PA does. Take notes. Ask questions about the practitioner's educational experience, their typical day at work, and their likes and dislikes about what they do. Realize that by allowing you to follow them around and by answering your questions, they are doing you a huge favor and they are taking time out of their day just for you. For this reason, you should always send a hand-written thank you note afterwards.

If you have made a good impression during your shadowing session, you may be able to ask the PA for a recommendation letter at some point. Try to express the desire for a recommendation letter sooner rather than later, as you want to be fresh in their mind. A good rule of thumb for recommendation letters is to initially follow-up in one week's time, and then send a reminder two weeks later. Remember, that practicing physician assistants must put the needs of their patients first, so they may forget your request or put it on the back burner if they are busy.

Be professional and courteous about the request, and offer to make it as easy for the PA as possible by providing them will all of the necessary information beforehand. For example, you may want to provide them with your resume (or a document with some brief information about your background and interests), so they have a better understanding of what your reasons are for wanting to become a PA. You should also provide them with the necessary envelopes (already addressed and stamped) if the provider needs to send it to a school or directly to the central application service for physician assistants.

The Value of Professional Organizations

Another great way to become a stronger applicant is to join a professional organization. Not only will you obtain a great deal of information about the profession by reading their newsletters or journals, but you can also network with other PAs in the organization. You will meet other students through the organization who are going through the same process you are. In addition, you can list your membership in the organization on your CASPA application. This is just one more method by which you can demonstrate your interest in the profession and express your desire to become a part of it.

In the first chapter, I mentioned that I served as student director of one of the PA organizations. While I was doing this, I constantly answered questions from Pre-PA students about applying to PA school. I even spent time critiquing personal statements from students before they applied to PA school. So, do not be afraid to contact the organization if you have questions or comments. Most organizations appreciate it when people are interested in learning more about them and the profession in general.

For starters, I would recommend joining your state PA organization and/or the AAPA. If you have a specific interest in a clinical specialty, you should join that particular organization. These organizations have programs already created for "Pre-PA" students like you, and student memberships are typically $50-$100. The cost may seem steep, so you should first decide if spending the money is worth it. Personally, I would say the cost is worth the opportunity to network and learn more about the profession, but I do know other physician assistants who might disagree with me. Based on your budget, decide what is best for you.

If you want to join one of these organizations, or simply want to find out more about them and read more about their activities, search for them online by the title of the organization or review the index in the back of the book. Here are just some of the varied, national PA organizations:

- American Academy of Physician Assistants ("AAPA")
- American Association of Surgical Physician Assistants ("AASPA")
- Association of Family Practice Physician Assistants ("AFPPA")
- Association of Physician Assistants in Cardiovascular Surgery ("APCVS")
- Society of Emergency Medicine Physician Assistants ("SEMPA")
- Association of Neurosurgical Physician Assistants ("ANSPA")
- Physician Assistants in Orthopaedic Surgery ("PAOS")

There are several others you may be interested in. The AAPA has a list of the constituent PA organizations. As of now, you can access this website online at: http://aapa.org/partners/constituent-organizations. (You can also review the Index of Physician Assistant Organizations at the end of the book).

Networking with other Pre-PA Students

No one will understand what you are going through better than someone who is also considering applying to PA school. Many universities now have "pre-PA clubs" that you can join to meet other students with your future career interests. I would encourage you to make friends with these people early on in your education. Spending more time with other focused individuals will help improve your chances of becoming a successful PA, seriously. As silly as it sounds, the old adage is true: surrounding yourself with like-minded individuals will keep you focused on your goal.

For this reason, you may also want to consider living in a pre-health or science-specific dormitory if one is offered at your university. Your pre-PA friends will enlighten you in many ways. For example, they might remind you of specific courses you should to take, when you should to take them, who might be the best professor to take a specific course with, they may share GRE resources with you, they may introduce you to a PA that will allow you to shadow him or her, they may have active discussions about the best and worst things about being a PA, etc. The ways in which spending time with other students pursing the profession will make you more competitive are endless—and not always obvious.

In addition to networking in-person (or, if you are a non-traditional student and do not have the ability to do this), use pre-PA resources online. There are several websites that allow pre-PA students to connect via the world-wide web. Below are just a few of what I believe are the best online resources for students interested in networking with other pre-PA students before PA school:

- **Physician Assistant ED**
  http://www.physicianassistanted.com

  - This website is dedicated to assisting pre-PA students. There are forums, regularly-scheduled chats with students and practicing physician assistants, blogs available for review, and many more resources for students. The site is well organized and very easy to use—I highly recommend checking it out, and I am a regular contributor.

- **The Physician Assistant Forum**
  http://www.physicianassistantforum.com

  - This website has been around for a long time, and has steadily filled with useful information. There are forums about everything you could possibly imagine related to entering PA school, being a PA student, and working as a PA. Many pre-PA students also use this site as a networking source.

- **Advance For Physician Assistants**
  http://www.advanceweb.com/nppa

  - This website provides a great deal of information about the profession and is updated frequently. There are PA student blogs and discussion boards that you can participate in.

- **The Student PA Path**
  http://www.TheStudentPAPath.com

  - This website is also dedicated to helping students gain admission to PA school. There are blogs available to review as well as options to utilize PA coaches. Use of the website requires a subscription, but the students who have used the program speak highly of it.

Healthcare Certification Courses

Another way you can make yourself a stronger applicant is by taking some relatively simple healthcare certification courses. Again, remember: whatever you can put on your CASPA application to positively present your commitment to the profession, you should. You can easily take a certification course in First Aid from the American Heart Association. You can also take a cardiopulmonary resuscitation ("CPR") course. Go to your local American Red Cross or American Heart Association to find out where and when the classes may be available. Earlier I mentioned taking a phlebotomy course. If you look online you can find weekend courses that provide a certification after only a few days of coursework. If you are just looking for a quick way to get the certificate and the training, this might be the route for you.

Keep in mind that the courses above may cost hundreds of dollars each, so you should determine how valuable you think this training might be before you spend the money. Think back, and do not forget any kind of health or wellness certification you have. I know people who have listed their yoga teaching certificates on their applications, as well as their personal training certificates. Including whatever certifications you have will make you stand out and will help give the PA program a better idea of who you are and what kind of healthcare provider you might be.

Pre-PA School Checklist

After reading through the information in this chapter, take careful stock in where you, as an applicant, stand today. Completing this chart will help you determine whether or not you are ready to apply to PA school. If you have marked off any items in the "no" category, you may want to consider waiting to apply to PA school until the following year so you can adequately prepare yourself.

Have you done these?	Yes	No	In Process
Taken Pre-Requisite Courses			
Shadowed a PA			
Worked or Volunteered in a Healthcare Setting			
Taken the GRE			
Made three Professional Contacts who would write Letters of Recommendation			
Achieved a desirable GPA			
Earned Bachelor's Degree (If PA School requires)			
Decided why you want to become a PA			
Researched the Schools you want to apply to			
Created a Support Network for yourself through friends and family			
Taken a Certification Course (CPR, First Aid, etc...)			
Considered how you will pay for PA School			

Deciding on Which Schools to Apply To

To date, there are 156 accredited physician assistant programs in the United States (and there will likely be more added to this list in the near future). Having a variety of programs to choose from is ideal; however, more options can make deciding where you might attend PA school more challenging. The most important part of selecting a school is your initial research. If you want to become a successful PA, you must be able to conduct research, and this is your first opportunity.

You have taken your first step by purchasing or reading this book, which will give you a foundation for beginning your search. Also, at the back of this book, I have included an index of every accredited PA program in the United States. This list should be a starting point for your search. Review the list of PA programs, highlight those you are interested in, and follow-up with even more research. Regardless of what I include in this book, there is no substitute for the time you will spend exploring the PA programs you identify as the most attractive to or suitable for you.

You should also examine programs by looking online to confirm whether a program is currently accredited. This is paramount, as it can impact your ability to become certified and work as a physician assistant. Those programs that are accredited have voluntarily undergone a rigorous review confirming their program meets the minimum Standards set in place for educational programs in the United States.[34] If a program is accredited, it is the program's responsibility to make sure that it is meeting these Standards.

To view the list of currently accredited PA programs, you can visit the Accreditation Review Commission on Education for the Physician Assistant ("ARC-PA") website at: http://www.arc-pa.org/acc _programs/index.html. On the website, the programs are listed in alphabetical order by state, and all of the programs' accreditation

---

[34] Accreditation Actions. ARC-PA Website. Available online at: http://www.arc-pa.org/acc_programs/acc_actions.html. Accessed on August 22, 2011.

information is provided. If you click on the link near each program you will be connected to that program's website.

There are occasionally broken links; if you find this to be the case, you should search for further information on the program directly and review their website (if there is no website, I advise you to reevaluate your choice of that specific program, and move onto the next on your list).   Do not be shy about contacting programs—many admissions professionals are eager to assist prospective students.

Another option, for those students without time to research each program, is a subscriber-based, on-line directory of PA programs. The Physician Assistant Education Association ("PAEA") provides a subscription website that provides pertinent program information. The cost for this service is currently $35 per subscription. The PAEA is a reputable PA organization, and for further information visit their website at: http://www.paeaonline.org.

The Physician Assistant ED website (http://www.physicianassistantED .com) has a comprehensive searchable PA program list as well. This site is very easy to use and has an extensive list of program information. You can view general information about PA programs, application deadlines and requirements, and contact information for free. If you become a subscriber of the website (which, as of now costs $3 per month), you will have access to further program search options, such as: each program's entrance requirements, costs associated with each program, host city information, chat rooms, and more.

Once you have reviewed the currently accredited programs, it is time to start making some initial decisions. Create a list of the programs you are interested in. At this point, it is fine if your list is lengthy—you will work on narrowing the list as you continue reading through this chapter. However, I would encourage you to begin thinking what issues might be especially important for you (and your family) throughout your PA education. For example, are you limited to a specific location and are you only interested in the programs near that location?   Or, are you looking for a program that will be the least expensive? Whatever your reason(s), decide which schools you are interested in (and I suggest you look at more than one program), and begin researching their programs more in-depth.

When I began searching for PA schools, I was not limited by anything but cost, and I was very open to traveling anywhere to go to school. For me, a lack of limitations made the process much more exciting because I had a huge initial number of programs to consider, and I was able to narrow it down to the top few that I thought were the best fit for me. I encourage you to first broaden your mental horizons. If you can go into the process with an open mind, you may find a program that you otherwise might have overlooked.

The best, first step to take to learn about a program is checking out their website. You can learn a number of things from your first visit, by asking a number of questions, such as:

- Is the website clear and easy to read?
- Is pertinent program information located on the site?
- Can I locate contact information on the website?
- Can I find out more about the faculty on the website?

If you can tell that the website has not been updated in a few years, it may also tell you something about the way the program operates. After checking out a program's website, you should start writing down key program information so you can compare schools. My personal advice is to make an excel spreadsheet (but you can write a grid out by hand) to compare program information. I have made a list of some of the most important items you should consider when selecting schools to apply to. I will discuss these items in greater detail following the list:

- Program Reputation
- Location
- Cost
- Type of Degree offered
- Program Curriculum
- Acceptance Rates
- Pre-requisite Requirements
- PANCE Pass Rate

- Drop-out Rates
- Housing Options
- Type of Rotations offered
- Travel Requirements during the program
- Shared Classes with other health students
- Opportunities to Study Abroad
- Opportunities to attend Advisory Sessions or Open Houses
- Opportunities to speak to former students

Reputation

You should definitely consider the school's reputation, but this should not be your only consideration. A school's reputation can be based on different items; however, the most important, for your application purposes, should be word of mouth and comparative studies. Pay attention to what you hear from PAs and other medical professionals who have graduated from the program, or those who have worked with PA graduates of the program. Word of mouth can help give you information about a school you otherwise may not have discovered.

Every year, U.S. News and World Report provides one issue that ranks graduate programs, including PA programs. While a great publication for a broad survey of PA programs, I suggest you use this guide only as part of your first consideration and take it with a grain of salt.

Unfortunately, like most reference books or sources, U.S. News and World Report has its flaws. Many schools do not participate in the U.S. News and World Report survey and are therefore excluded from the rankings. For instance, the 2007 survey only included 73 of the accredited PA programs (and there were more than 139 accredited programs at the time). I have no doubt that the schools listed are some of the best programs in the country, but I do believe that there are other excellent programs that were not included in the report because they did not participate.

In 2010, physician assistant educators published an article highlighting indicators that may be better-suited to rank PA programs.[35] The article suggests there are indicators overlooked by the U.S. News and World Report survey that may be important to consider when ranking PA programs. The authors suggest some additional items that should be included in ranking systems, including the program's 5-year PANCE scores, graduation or attrition rates, student-to-faculty ratios, full-time vs. part-time faculty ratios, the program's accreditation length granted, and the degrees offered by the program. The rankings change dramatically when these items are used to compare PA programs.

But, ultimately, it is up to you to decide how you feel about a given program's reputation. Use the items mentioned above to guide you, but use your gut instincts to help you determine whether or not a program is "good enough" for you.

Location

I think for most people location is one of the most important factors. If you have a family, you may only be able to look at a few of the programs that are closest to where you and your family are living. In fact, that is a typical reason why people apply to certain programs— simply because it is the only program close by. Do not feel bad if that is the predicament you are in; instead, consider yourself lucky to have a family support system to help get you through PA school.

Your local or regional school also likely has many practicing alumni in your area, and this may help with future shadowing experiences or job searches. However, if you are like I was, and are not glued to a specific location, you should feel free to explore all types of programs to really see which one might best meet your needs.

If you are not limited by location, you should try to decide which type of setting you desire. Do you want to live in a big city for a few years, or would you prefer to be in a smaller town that is primarily supported

---

[35] Van Rhee, J., Davanzo, M. A Novel Approach to Ranking Physician Assistant Programs. *Journal of Physician Assistant Education.* 2010;21(4):30-36.

by the local university. Do you want to drive your own car or rely on public transportation? Remember, that city living tends to be a bit more costly when compared to otherwise comparable rural settings.

Another consideration is the weather. As silly as it sounds, you should think carefully about how a significant change in climate might affect you. If you have spent your entire life living in Florida, where temperatures are high year-round, moving to a setting with long-cold winters may present new challenges that you did not expect. (Alternatively, the idea of a long-cold winter could also be appealing to you). Make sure you at least consider how a school's climate might impact you personally—as this will alter your outlook throughout the year and likely your study habits.

Cost

For most people, the cost of the program is extremely important. Some programs offer in-state tuition, which makes the programs much more affordable and lessens your debt load. Private institutional programs may cost much more when compared to public schools. Be honest about how much you can afford initially. If you are like most students, you will want to know how much student loan debt you will have after you have finished the program. I can personally tell you paying off student loan debt is *very* difficult, and I guarantee most of my PA friends and colleagues feel the same way. Most physician assistant students do require student loans and can eventually pay them off, but putting half of your salary towards your student loan payment each month is not fun. The cost associated with PA school can hang over your head for years, if not decades, so consider the cost of school carefully from the beginning.

Type of Degree Offered

Another important issue when considering programs is deciding which "degree" you want to obtain. Most PA programs have converted to master's degree programs, or are in the process of converting to a master's degree. However, there are still some programs that only offer a certificate of completion, and others that offer a bachelor's degree or an associate's degree instead. There is no right or wrong here; if the program is accredited, you will be able to sit for the Physician Assistant National Certifying Exam ("PANCE") and become a certified PA. You should decide which degree is appropriate for you and cross off those that do not provide you with the degree you are most interested in. Just know that while the degree should not matter for clinical practice, it may affect other possible future work paths, such as teaching or pursuing other types of higher education.

Curriculum

You must consider each program's curriculum. How much time is spent on the didactic portion versus the clinical portion of the program? Which of the two are you more comfortable with? Do you personally believe you will benefit from a longer period of time in the classroom (the didactic portion) or from more time taking care of patients (the clinical portion)? Some programs are evenly balanced with 12 months of didactic training and 12 months of clinical training; however, some programs provide much more time in the classroom than on the patient floors. You should try to determine which may be better for you and better match your learning style or needs.

When looking at a program's curriculum, you should also make sure there is a cadaver lab for anatomy classes. More and more programs are getting away from the hands-on experience you get as a student in the cadaver lab, but I believe it is vital to learning the human body and to functioning as a successful PA in the future. A CD-ROM with pictures of the human body simply does not compare to the experience you get actually dissecting the human body in a cadaver lab. I speak from my own experience, and I have confirmed this with physicians and PAs I have worked with.

Research what the program requires for graduation. Many PA programs require students to complete a master's thesis or a final project of some type. Some programs encourage students to participate in research opportunities within the university or hospital system, while others do not offer this option. Each program has created their own graduation requirements, but exploring what those are may be important—especially if you have a desire to publish work in the future or get experience working on a clinical trial.

There are other aspects of a program's curriculum I would suggest you explore. Some programs include additional coursework that may enhance your ability to successfully pass the PANCE and work as a PA in the future. While these are not required courses at many programs, I think having instruction in the following topics may be useful for solidifying your basic science foundation: genetics, nutrition, biochemistry, and statistics.

Acceptance Rate

Consider each school's acceptance rate. You should be able to contact the school to find out the average GPA and the total number of applicants, and you can consult my research in the index of PA programs located at the end of this book. This will help you determine whether or not the program is "within reach" for you. Obviously, if you have a 2.8 GPA and the school's acceptance average was 3.6, you may want to reconsider applying there. Or, if the school typically receives 1,000 applicants and only accepts 30 students per class, you know you are going to have to be an exceptional applicant if you are going to stand a chance at being admitted. Determine this before you apply, and you may save on application fees—as well as potential heartache if your first choice school was too far out of reach.

Pre-Requisite Requirements

You should determine what pre-requisite coursework is required by the PA program. If you were an English major as an undergraduate, you may have taken very few science courses. It is likely you are going to want to find a program that requires fewer science pre-requisites because you will not want to take pre-requisites for PA school for an additional 2-3 years (unless you have unlimited time and money). However, if you were a pre-PA or pre-med in undergrad, this may not matter at all.

Also, keep in mind that most schools favor coursework taken at a university when compared to a community college. They also favor "upper level" science courses when compared to introductory science courses (for example, Biochem 300 is a stronger choice than Biochem 101). If you have taken all of your science courses at a community college because it was less expensive, you might be at a disadvantage. Contact the school and find out if they rank their students based on this criteria. Some schools favor the quality of the coursework, while other schools value the grade you received in the course compared to where the course was taken or what level the course was listed at. This is important information that may have a significant impact on your chances for acceptance into your chosen program.

When I was teaching, I did not believe where a student took the course impacted his or her ability to successfully learn the material. Mastering content is the purpose of taking a course, and this can be demonstrated by achieving a top grade in the course, independent of where the course was taken. If you received top grades at a community college, I think it is fair to argue that your knowledge level is likely comparable to someone who took the course at a large university.

Achieving high grades at a large university may demonstrate an ability to succeed without as much one-on-one assistance from a professor, but this does not mean that the student did not require additional tutoring or use of the university's vast teaching and learning resources. The point I am trying to make is this: if you received a high grade in a course, chances are you have garnered an adequate foundation of the material. Unless the PA applicant pool is full of exceptional students, having taken a few science courses at a community college (and done well in them) should not impact your ability to obtain admission to a program significantly.

PANCE Pass Rate

You should be able to find out the Physician Assistant National Certifying Examination ("PANCE") pass rates for the past few years. As I mentioned before, the PANCE is the certifying exam that PAs must take in order to become credentialed and actually practice as a PA. The "PANCE pass rate" simply refers to how many students passed the examination the first time. Many schools will advertise this on their website, but others may decline simply because their scores were low. All things being equal, if you are considering a specific school, find out that school's PANCE pass rate, especially the first-time pass rate. The rate it is indicative as to how well the school prepares their students to take the national exam and pass it, as well as how well they are training their students to practice as PAs professionally.

If I found out that many students failed the national certifying exam, I am not sure that I would want to attend that program. Your goal is to get the best quality education. Your secondary goal is then to pass the exam after you finish school. Therefore, you want to select a school that has a high PANCE first-time pass rate. Usually, if a school has one or two students fail the exam (which is common—it is a difficult exam), the rate will still be at or above 90%. If a school's first-time pass rate is lower than that, try to find out why. The vast majority of students graduating from a well-run program should be passing the exam.

Drop-Out Rates

You should also ask how many students typically begin the program, and how many end up dropping out of the program. If there are more than one or two students that drop out each year, find out why. Is the program too difficult? Does the program allow students who may not be appropriate for PA school to attend the program simply to "get their money" before failing them out?   I do not believe the latter is true of any program, but if you notice a significant number of drop-outs, you should definitely be concerned as to why the program is losing students. Do not put yourself in the position to be a borderline student that may be left behind by a program.

Keep in mind that it is common for one or two students to get left behind each year. While PA programs try to prevent this as they want their students to be successful, some students may not make the cut academically or may need to de-matriculate for personal reasons.

Housing Options

If you are looking at attending a school outside of your home-town, you should find out if the school offers student housing. If available, how much will student housing cost you? If student housing is unavailable, what is the cost of an apartment in the area? Remember to include this in the budget you completed in the previous section of the book.

If you are married or have a family, you will want to determine what the options are available for you and those people who will be living with you. Some PA programs offer extensive residential housing options that include reduced-rate apartments for students with families. Others do not, and you will need to seek out what an apartment in the area might cost.

When seeking out apartment rates, keep proximity to school in mind. You will likely be spending a great deal of time on campus and will want to live close to school (within walking distance is ideal). So, when exploring housing options, try to avoid seeking out apartment rents in a town that is 30 miles away (unless you have a very good reason for this).

Types of Rotations Offered

You should find out what types of rotations are available. If you know you want to work in a particular specialty, for example, cardiothoracic surgery, find out how much time (if any) you will be able to spend participating in rotations related to your interests. Will you get elective rotations that you can choose yourself? If so, how many, and what is the duration of each rotation? Will you need to travel a great distance to obtain this experience?

PA programs will provide you with a solid foundation by requiring you to participate in several primary care rotations throughout the duration of PA school. That being said, schools in rural areas may not have access to full-length clinical rotations in a few areas of medicine (such as long-term care, psychiatry, or obstetrics and gynecology). This does not bother most students as they obtain adequate exposure to these areas of medicine throughout the duration of their education. But, if you have a specific interest in working in one of these specialties in the future, you may want to find out if the PA program offers full-length rotations in all of the areas of medicine you desire.

Remember, rotation sites for PA students are not always easy to secure, especially if the program is competing with area medical schools. You may find that you are required to complete rotations with several other students, some of which may be nurse practitioner or medical students.

Some students find this desirable and others do not. Try to decide if the idea of rural rotations or working with multiple students impacts you and your learning goals in any way.

Travel Requirements

Will you be required to travel during your rotations? Some programs are set up so the didactic portion of the program is completed in its entirety at one site, and then the clinical rotations are conducted all over the state. This occurs because the program may need to rely on additional medical facilities to help meet the educational needs of all of their students.

Most programs are very up-front about this during the application and interview process as they want their students to be well-informed of any potential driving (or relocating) that may be required during the program. If you are hoping to stay in one particular area because of your family, this may cause problems. In rural areas, traveling offsite (and sometimes very far offsite) is quite common. Keep potential family problems in this area to a minimum by finding out if you will be required to travel for rotations before you apply.

Shared Classes?

You should find out if the program has another graduate health program at the same site. Sometimes institutions with medical schools, physical therapy programs, and PA schools require all of those students to take some of their classes together. This is typically frowned upon because the educational programs have different learning goals, but it can and does happen at some schools.

I have known many students who have actually enjoyed integrated classrooms, but others who found it quite bothersome. Find out if your program does this and consider whether this is something that may lessen your interest. PA school is difficult enough as is. You do not wish to be distracted, or to have program glitches lessen your interest in the curriculum.

Opportunities to Travel Abroad

Today, PA students can participate in rotations overseas during their clinical rotations. If this is something you are interested in, you should find out if the program offers opportunities like this, or other more novel approaches to teaching or clinical experiences. Some programs may have organized rotation sites abroad, and others may require the student to set up the rotation independently. Explore this option if it is something you are passionate about and wish to include in your journey to becoming a PA.

Advisory Sessions

You should find out if the program has an open house or an advisory session. **If so, you should absolutely go!** These sessions are often great opportunities to meet the faculty and talk to current students. You can also tour the facilities while you are there. You should look at the classrooms and the labs. You will be spending a lot of time in these rooms as a student—do they look comfortable and well-lit, or are they dark and musty? Participating in an open house or advisory session is one of the best ways to really get a personal feel for the school and to determine whether or not it is right for you.

If you attend an open house or an advisory session, you should also send a thank you note directed to those members of the faculty who took time to answer your questions and show you around campus—so remember to get business cards or contact information at the session. If you do decide to send a note or follow-up e-mail, remember to keep it simple, professional, and to the point. Your goal is to express your gratitude and to possibly make yourself stand out just a little bit more. While some universities do not keep the letters due to space limitations, others will retain them in a file with your application.

Opportunities to Speak with Students

You should find out if there are opportunities to speak with current or former students. After connecting with a current or former student, you may learn things about the program that either discourage you, or further inspire you to attend. Current and former students of the program are some of the best resources to find out the "scoop" about the program. They will likely tell you all the good and all the bad because they are not obligated to sell the program, whereas school administrators are paid to sugar-coat their programs.

What is Missing?

After you have made your list and reviewed each school's website, find out what information is missing from the list and contact the schools directly to complete your research. These questions will elicit pertinent information that the program should be able to supply you with. I would try contacting each program via e-mail first, and if you do not get a response within a few days, then follow-up with them by phone.

Programs are used to being contacted about these issues, and most have administrative staff in place to take care of answering questions about the program. But, I do urge you to try not to be too annoying when following up with questions. You do not want to be the "annoying prospect who calls every day" with questions—that will get you the type of name recognition you do not want! Take the time to think about your questions, and write them down before contacting the program. Remember to first make sure you have explored the website and that the information is unavailable before you contact them. Call once with all of your collected questions, rather than multiple times.

The bottom line is simple: do your research. Once you have determined which schools meet your personal preferences, you can narrow your selections down and begin the application process.

How to Apply to PA School

Applying to PA school represents the first step in a truly life-changing decision. And your reward (once you have made the decision to apply, and have confirmed that you have completed the necessary pre-requisites for admission), is that you get to begin the tedious application process. And, if you thought being an actual PA student was going to be the only difficult part, welcome to the admissions process. Not surprisingly, the application process will take a great deal of work as well.

Central Application Service for Physician Assistants

In order to apply to most accredited PA schools, you will use the Central Application Service for Physician Assistants ("CASPA"). CASPA is a system that allows you to submit all of your information online in a single-application format. Once CASPA receives all of your information, it is then forwarded on to the programs to which you are applying. This system streamlines the application process, making it relatively easy for both you and the schools you are applying to.

To begin the application process, you will need to register as a user on the CASPA website. As of now, the CASPA website is: https://portal.caspaonline.org. Even if you are not quite ready to begin an application, I would encourage you to register as a user. This will allow you to check out the site, see what information you will need to eventually enter, and give you a head start on compiling that information. And, once you have registered to use the website, you can begin the application process at anytime within the specified time frame (generally from April of the current year to March of the next year).

Currently, there are 156 accredited U.S. PA programs, and 148 of those programs use the CASPA application system.[36] That means that there are still a few programs (but less than 10) that use their own proprietary applications. Before you begin entering your information into the CASPA website, check to see if your school choices use the central application service, or if they use their own applications. You may need to apply online using the CASPA system for some schools, and fill out separate applications to for schools that do not use the CASPA.

The most important thing I can tell you about applying to PA school is to **apply early**. If at all possible, beat the application deadline by at least a month. The PA school application process is lengthy, and is built on prior actions, step-by-step. If you send your application in late, you will not be considered for admission, no matter how attractive a candidate you are. The sooner the school receives your application, the sooner the school can begin evaluating you, and (hopefully) admitting you to their upcoming PA class.

Entering the information into the CASPA system is very time consuming and people oftentimes do not realize how taxing the process can be. The sooner you start entering information, the more time you get to focus on the rest of your application materials as deadlines begin to approach. Just as you will need to be organized when you are a physician assistant student, you will need to be organized when using the central application service for PAs. Your first step should be to start a "CASPA folder," in which you will organize and collect all of the information you need for your application. Your folder can be digital if you decide to keep scanned records of the necessary items. This folder should include at least the following:

- Transcripts from the institutions you have attended (official copies will be sent directly to the CASPA, but you may and should obtain student copies for your records)

---

[36] Accreditation Review Commission on Education for the Physician Assistant, Inc. Program Data. Available online at: http://www.arc-pa.org/acc_programs/program_data.html. Accessed on August 22, 2011.

- Your standardized test scores (official copies will be sent directly to the CASPA, but you may and should obtain student copies for your own records)
- Records for any certifications you have obtained (and certainly those you mention on your application)
- Your employment history
- Your health-related experience and/or direct patient contact information
- Your community service information
- Contact information for the people who will write your letters of recommendation

Once you have collected these items, carefully organize them in your CASPA folder. You should then create a timeline for yourself. If you know, for example, that the school of your choice has an application deadline of October 1st, work backwards and plan to submit your application by September 1st. This will also help you make a timeline detailing when you will enter the necessary information into the CASPA system, as well as when you will need to order your transcripts and obtain your letters of recommendation. It cannot be emphasized enough that you need to be organized in order to finish everything related to the application process in a timely manner.

The central application for physician assistants is fairly user friendly; however, if you are not comfortable with computers, you may have a more difficult time using the program. To begin, read the CASPA section titled, "Before Applying." You may also wish to review the "Instructions" and "FAQ" sections before you get started.

Once you are comfortable with the website, click on "My Application" and begin entering in the appropriate information. The site is "secure," so you should feel safe entering personal information, such as your social security number and contact information. Write down your username and password on the inside of your CASPA folder cover so you do not forget them. You will be accessing this site frequently, so you want to make sure you can always log in properly.

Begin filling in the contact information, and carefully complete each section. Make sure you enter the information as accurately as possible.

Enter all of the schools you attended, and all of the grades you received (even the not-so-good ones; every year there is always at least one student that does not heed this advice). Under the "Additional Information" section, there are questions about whether or not you have ever been in legal or academic trouble. You must be honest when answering these questions. If you have been on academic probation or have been convicted of a misdemeanor, you need to include this information.

There is a section that allows you to provide an explanation as to what circumstances may have lead to the issue at hand. **Be advised: You must not lie or exaggerate on this application—do not jeopardize your career before it even begins.** The application material will be crosschecked against your official transcripts and supplied documents, and falsifying any information could potentially exclude you from the application process—or could derail your studies, or even your career, years later.

While entering information on the CASPA, there are a few areas that ask you to explain your "duties." Try to keep your explanations as brief as you can. The amount of space you have to write is limited to approximately 110 words, and you cannot exceed this limit as your writing will get cut off mid-sentence.

Your Narrative or Personal Statement

The narrative or personal statement is another section of the application in which the length of your writing is limited. Currently, the central application service allows you submit a narrative that is a maximum of 625 words or 5,000 characters. This is approximately one page in Microsoft Word using Times New Roman 12 point font, single-spaced.

If you are using the CASPA system, your personal statement should "describe your motivation towards becoming a PA." And, you must describe this motivation in approximately 625 words or less. I can tell you from personal experience, limiting your personal statement is not easy. You will have to write and edit, then re-write, and re-edit.

As part of your editing process, have several people read your essay to make sure it flows well and is grammatically correct. **Read it aloud at least once.** You want to make sure you have created the perfect description of why you want to become a physician assistant. I would recommend reading the instructions for the narrative carefully, as formatting issues may occur when copying and pasting your essay into the appropriate section on the CASPA website. Once you have copied and pasted your narrative into the CASPA website, make sure it looks exactly how you want it to look.

Before beginning your essay, take a moment to consider who you are and what you have done thus far in your life. To get you started, I have outlined a few questions you should ask yourself. Take the time to write down your answers to each of these questions—doing so may help give you ideas for your essay topic, and can help if you find yourself stuck.

- What initially sparked your decision to become a physician assistant?
- What healthcare experiences have you had (paid or volunteer), and what have you learned from each?
- What jobs have you held, and what have you learned from each?
- What volunteer experiences have you had, and what have you learned from each?
- Have you had any personal or family medical experiences that influenced your decision to become a physician assistant? If so, what were they?
- What have you learned through your shadowing experiences with PAs?
- What is unique about you? (Do you have any hobbies or talents?)
- If you applied to physician assistant school before and were rejected, what did you learn? And, what have you done since that time to improve your chances of being accepted?
- What are you currently doing to make yourself a stronger applicant?
- What are you currently doing to make yourself a better, future PA?

- Have you had any unique patient experiences that have inspired you?
- Have you participated in any type of research? If so, what did you learn from it?
- Have you traveled abroad, if so what did you learn from your experience?

After answering all of these questions, you should be ready to start your essay. Some of the hard work will already be done: simply review all of the information you have written down and see where it leads you.

When I was teaching, the most successful personal essays I reviewed were "from the heart." These essays are usually simple in nature, and tend to have a theme or a story about what inspired the applicant to become a PA. It is ok to talk about your academic history and anything unique about you (perhaps you are a concert pianist or a college athlete). But you should make your essay both a reflection of who you are now and who you want to become as a PA.

As with any essay, it is important to have both a strong start and finish to your essay. And, always be as clear as you possibly can. You do not need to use complicated words in your essay; you just need to write in a way that allows people to understand exactly what you are trying to say.

Demonstrating your passion to become a PA is imperative in your personal statement. Many times, applicants express a desire to work in "healthcare" or "medicine." Using vague statements like this does not convey your knowledge of the profession or your desire to become a part of it. If you make it clear that you have shadowed physician assistants and are certain that being a family practice or surgical PA is the career for you, your essay is more likely to stand out.

If you are still having trouble with how to write the essay, you may wish to consider going to the writing center at a local college or university. Oftentimes, colleges have staff members who can help students with writing assignments or projects for free.

It is extremely important that you actually write your own essays. While you may have others help you edit your essay, make sure the material you write and submit is actually your own. Plagiarism, or any other uncredited use of another's words or ideas, are serious offenses and oftentimes have severe consequences.

Many PA programs may ask you to write additional impromptu essays during your interview in order to compare the sample with your actual CASPA narrative. If your essay is really good (or striking in some fashion), admissions staff will enter specific phrases into search engines or submit them to school plagiarism services. Write your own essay and do not plagiarize; it simply is not worth the risk involved.

To help you get an idea of what a narrative or personal statement should look like, I have included some examples of successful essays— each of these students was accepted to the PA program of their choice. Also, these essays were all entered into the CASPA system, and each is less than 5,000 characters. You may like some but not others, but remember that these were all "winning essays," such that the students who wrote them were accepted to a PA program. Pick one, or several, whose style seems comfortable, and try writing your first draft with that style in mind. But, of course, these essays are here to help you generate your own ideas, not to copy other individuals' material.

Essay One:

> Mrs. Weippert, my biology teacher in the 10th grade, sparked
> my interest in medicine in two ways, with her enthusiasm for
> teaching the life sciences in a "hands-on" approach and by her
> personal struggle with cancer. The end of the year project in
> Biology was to dissect a cat. This "hands-on" activity deepened
> my appreciation for the complexity of the mammalian body. I
> could only imagine the magnitude of detail that composed the
> human body. Shortly after the cat dissections, Mrs. Weippert
> was readmitted into the hospital for her struggle with breast
> cancer. During the summer, Mrs. Weippert passed away. This
> experience made me realize the frailty of our body that supports
> life. As a result of her death and the knowledge of Biology she

taught me, I knew that a career in the medical field would be one that I would find rewarding.

In high school, I worked hard for my grades in pursuit of a career in the medical field and I was rewarded with the honor of being Valedictorian of my class. However, limited in the amount of science preparation I received in high school, I struggled in my first few years of college. I struggled with learning at the college level, more specifically only in my science courses such as Cell and Molecular Biology and Organic Chemistry. I chose to retake these courses with the same professors I had first taken the courses with as a way to prove to myself and to my professors the degree of my perseverance. Although only having had limited experience in the medical field, I continued along the pre-medical track trying to figure out where in the medical field I belonged.

My decision to become a physician assistant arose from two separate experiences during the summer of 2006. Working as a nurse's aide and job shadowing influenced my decision. In May of 2006, I obtained a job working as a nurse's aide in a dementia care senior living facility. My duties consisted of taking vitals, passing medications, applying bandages, showering residents, and helping with tasks such as eating and ambulating. The tasks I performed allowed me to personally connect with the residents which I found especially rewarding.

Working in this type of medical setting also showed me the importance of teamwork in the medical field. On one specific day, the residents were to be examined by their primary care physician. The physician filed through the residents never speaking and only checking heart rates. For the fifteen second exam each resident was charged the full exam rate. The runny nose and the rash went unnoticed. I was filled with disgust. I saw first-hand how physicians no longer work on their own terms. During a Health Economics course, I learned that most physicians are ruled by an insurer who tells them how many patients they must see a day. After witnessing this first-hand, I knew I did not want to work in a career in which the human connection was lost due to time constraints and heavy influenced placed on making money. In order to be certain that I did not want to become a physician I decided to also job shadow during the summer.

During my job shadowing experience, I was faced with the facts about the life of a physician. I learned about high insurance costs and their busy schedules which limits the time they are able to spend with their families. What I learned about being a physician put into prospective what I personally needed out of a career. I wanted a career that would allow me the ability to diagnose and treat, have time to spend with my family, and have the opportunity for variety within my career.

I began talking with people who worked in the medical field and many suggested the career of a physician assistant. Liz, a physician assistant in a town nearby my college deeply impressed me with her knowledge, compassion, and enthusiasm for her job. From other shadowing opportunities I learned about the versatility of the career and the ability to change specialties without further schooling. Working under a physician has its benefits. During difficult diagnoses the physician is available for consultation. The ability to work as a team appeals to me much more so than working independently. The role of a physician assistant is one that defines exactly what I want to do within the medical field.

I believe that the struggles I encountered in college helped me to mature, and I do not regard them as mistakes, they were learning experiences. My personal experiences in 2006, reassured me that a career in the medical field would be gratifying and one in which I would be able to demonstrate my compassion for others. The qualities that I saw in the physician assistants that I shadowed I saw in myself. I know that being a physician assistant is what I want and it is where I am needed.

Essay Two:

My siblings and I are the first generation in my family to go to college. Our parents worked hard to furnish our basic needs and ensure a valuable education that provided us with the opportunity to do something useful with our lives. My dad spent many hours working overtime at factory jobs to enable us to afford higher goals, so we would not have to do the same. Being adopted from Korea, I am especially grateful to my parents for giving me a new life. Their philosophy of hard work and determination has motivated me to do something meaningful with my life.

Still, it was from my grandparents that I learned the meaning of compassion and goodwill. Always devoted to helping others, my grandparents volunteered at the hospital, donated money to charities, volunteered as a fireman, and donated over thirty gallons of blood. They stimulated me to look into a career that benefited others. I researched all of my options dutifully, yet it was difficult deciding what path because I wanted to make the right decision.

However, when my grandmother was diagnosed suddenly with cancer and died soon after, I knew that I wanted to be involved in healthcare. For those last days of her life, I took care of her to make her last days as comfortable as possible. It was one of the hardest things I have ever done, but it was also one of the most rewarding. I was able to take care of my grandmother, just like she had done for me throughout my life. This life changing event inspired me.

Ever since I was little I had wanted, like many children, to become a doctor. After researching though, I knew I wanted to be a physician assistant because of their phenomenal and growing reputation in the world of medicine as respected workers who get to focus primarily on the patients and not on the politics. I became determined to achieve my goal of becoming a physician assistant.

I know that I have the strength, compassion, and determination to become a competent PA. This past year has really tested me to see if it was the right choice. Along with taking my regular classes, I held four jobs, took summer classes and was co-captain on my college cheerleading team, all while maintaining a GPA of 3.7. I was accepted into the health professions honor society, Alpha Epsilon Delta and accepted into Mortarboard which recognizes senior college students for their achievements in leadership, scholarship, and service. My job as a Certified Nurse's Aide in long-term care has shown me that I am strong enough physically and emotionally to cope with disease and death. I love working with the residents and trying to make their lives happy and purposeful.

My motivation to be a PA has come mostly from my family's influences of selflessness and hard work. I have a passion for wanting to heal others and if given the opportunity, I will help them altruistically so they can continue making lasting memories with their families and friends. Hopefully, I can make a difference in people's lives just as others have done for me and my family.

Essay Three:

Upon graduating from high school in 2002, I chose a nontraditional career path by serving in the Navy as an aviation electronics technician for four and a half years. During that time frame, I learned to work under large amounts of stress, pay strict attention to detail, and to function as an effective team member. Upon my honorable discharge in December 2006, I planned to pursue a career as a commercial aviation pilot since I had earned my private pilot's license a few years earlier. However, I quickly learned that this was a poor career choice for me because of its job placement.

As a result, I started looking at careers in the health care field because I have always had an interest in this area. Initially, I started as a Clinical Laboratory Science major when I enrolled in college in the spring of 2007. That major seemed enticing because it combined two of my favorite subjects: Biology and Chemistry. However, as I gained a better understanding of this career field, I realized that it did not suit me well. I still wanted to pursue a major in the health care field but wanted the deep satisfaction that comes from being able to directly help people. After doing some research and meeting with my academic advisor, I decided to focus my career goals on becoming a physician assistant. The prospect of becoming a physician was unappealing given the large time and monetary commitment it would require. However, being a physician assistant would encompass my favorite academic subjects, allow me to treat and diagnose diseases, and enable me to help people.

I changed my major to Biological Sciences during that first semester and decided to shadow the physician assistants at the local primary care clinic once the semester had ended. This shadowing experience would help ensure that being a physician assistant was something that I truly wanted. I was able to shadow two family practice physician assistants and another that worked in orthopedics.

During my shadowing experience, I was very surprised with the amount of autonomy the physician assistants had. They often worked very independently, but would work closely with a physician on more complex cases. The orthopedic physician assistant would manage his time by seeing patients in the clinic but also acted as the first assistant during many of the surgical cases. Also, many of the patients I met remarked at how much they enjoyed being seen by physician assistants because they tended to spend more time with them and seemed more personable. It was also gratifying to see the tight knit bond that was formed between the physician assistants and the patients.

These observations during my shadowing experience only served to reinforce my goal of becoming a physician assistant. Given my strong academic background, diverse work experience, compassionate nature, and strong desire to become a physician assistant, I feel I would be an excellent addition to your program.

Essay Four:

As a practicing certified (and licensed) athletic trainer, I have spent my career specializing in the prevention, recognition, management and rehabilitation of injuries that result from physical activity. Working under the direction of licensed physicians and in cooperation with other health care professionals has given me a solid understanding of how to work as part of a health care team. My work experience has helped me understand how each medical professional plays a significant role in providing sound health care to our communities. Physician assistants are an integral part of today's team based health care system, and I believe my academic and professional experience has provided me with a solid foundation on which to build a career as a physician assistant.

I see many of the qualities that I posses mirrored in the physician assistants that I have come in contact with. I am honest, compassionate, knowledgeable and I posses a strong desire to help others. As a physician assistant, I want to use my skills and attributes to help others live a healthy lifestyle. I am passionate about health care, and I want to help others achieve soundness of mind and body, so they can be active and live a happy and fulfilling life.

I have pursued health care as a career because helping others has always been very natural for me. My experience as an athletic trainer has been extremely gratifying and rewarding. However, at this point in my life I feel that I am ready to broaden my scope as a health care professional. I want to practice the kind of medicine where compassion, personal caring and medical excellence are the cornerstones of success. This is exactly what physician assistants do!

As a physician assistant, I will enjoy greater autonomy, along with treating a broader population of patients with varying types of conditions. I like to be challenged, and I enjoy the challenge of recognizing an injury or condition, devising a plan of treatment, and then guiding that person through the process of healing, physically, emotionally and psychologically. I am ready to take my medical knowledge to the next level and there is no challenge better suited for me than becoming a physician assistant.

Medicine fascinates me. I am amazed by the complexity of the human body, and the delicate balance between wellness and illness and how to maintain it. I want to become more of a participant in the management of peoples' health care concerns. Through job shadowing and working professionally with physicians and physician assistants, I have reaffirmed that becoming a physician assistant is the career I want to pursue. I work hard, study hard and I believe in my abilities. This is something I've wanted to do for a long time. I am ready for this challenge.

Essay Five:

I was first introduced to medicine while I was working as a student athletic trainer for my undergraduate college's sports teams. The demographic of patients being young, active, and compliant with treatment protocols made the concept of athletic training appealing to me. Although I learned a great deal from the profession, it left me wanting to learn more from a medical standpoint.

In the role of student athletic trainer, I got the opportunity to observe our team's orthopedic physician, along with his physician assistant, who was a former athletic trainer himself. After being fortunate enough to observe them perform a rotator cuff and meniscal repair surgery, I was hooked.

I want to be given more responsibility in the medical field, and to test my skills at a higher level of medicine. I yearn to be involved in the progress of patients from the early stages of their medical history, to ordering and interpreting diagnostic tests, and finally, in performing or assisting with surgical procedures and recovery. The professionalism, organization, and respect the field of physician assistant possesses are something to marvel at. It is my impression that there is no room for complacency in this field, and I have the drive and energy to succeed and excel in it. There are the stringent guidelines of maintaining 100 CME hours every two years, along with the requirement of passing the re-certification test every six years.

I find myself motivated by the growing need for physician assistants as managed care organizations look to mid-level practitioners to lower the cost of healthcare for an increasingly dependent "baby boomer" population. I also appreciate that there is freedom to move through different fields in medicine while in the role of a physician assistant.

After working in a hospital and hearing from a variety of patients about the connections they have made with their physician assistants, it makes me realize the importance and value of their jobs, and also makes me want to be a part of a team that can help people. I want to be challenged everyday while earning a living, and I feel that the occupation of physician assistant would more than reciprocate that ambition.

Essay Six:

A child's parents came up to me the day they were finally able to take their son home from the children's hospital and said, "Thank you so much for reading and drawing with our son these past few months. We truly believe it accelerated his healing and we were also able to enjoy lunch breaks and run errands." Since applying to the physician assistant (PA) program last year, I have had many positive experiences like this one that have reinforced my desire to work full-time in patient care as a PA. My involvement with patient cases in the microbiology lab, PA shadowing experiences, children's hospital experiences, and work as a personal care attendant have all strengthened my passion for a career as a PA.

My initial interest in becoming a PA began while working as a medical technologist where I help physicians with case studies. Often they inform me of a patient's history and we discuss options for antibiotic treatment based on susceptibility results.

Analyzing case studies became my favorite part of this job and I desired to work more directly with patients.

I arranged a shadowing experience with a PA in the gynecology clinic, and observed her examining and educating patients on health topics such as the new HPV vaccine. This was appealing since I have always enjoyed teaching. Throughout my schooling I have tutored my classmates and in college I was a student teaching assistant for a bacteriology lab. I became very excited about becoming a PA. Here was a career where I could combine my love for helping people, medicine, and teaching!

Next, I shadowed two PAs during patient rounds on the transplant unit at the hospital. I observed how doctors, PAs, nurses, and pharmacists work as a team to provide integrated patient care. In my additional experiences as a volunteer and personal care attendant I have learned that patient care can be both challenging and rewarding. Volunteering in a children's hospital unit is challenging at times, such as when a child refuses to end playtime to take medication. It is extremely rewarding to be a personal care attendant for a woman with spinal muscular atrophy. My drive to become a PA increased when I saw how my efforts directly impacted her day-to-day successes in school. While I have been her attendant she has completed law school and is now a practicing attorney.

I greatly desire to become a PA because this career would integrate my passions: medicine, patient care, teaching, teamwork, and critical-thinking. The flexibility of changing specialties is also very attractive. In preparation for starting a PA program, I recently completed a two semester course in Anatomy and Physiology. This fall I am enrolled in a Certified Nursing Assistant (CNA) course and will become CNA certified this December. I am dedicated to work thereafter as a CNA in order to further prepare me for success as a PA.

Essay Seven:

My desire to become a physician assistant is derived from a wealth of fortunate coincidences:

First, my work as a student in the healthcare field has provided me many unique opportunities to participate in patient education while I prepared to apply to physician assistant school. I also believe my desire to enter into the PA field stems from several specific experiences, which include personal interactions with physician assistants, working with patients in various settings, the challenge of critically thinking and forming rational intervention plans, and being part of the maturation of healthcare as it continues to improve patient care.

Second, as a patient, I have been impressed by the professionalism and care provided by physician assistants. I began exploring the profession when I was an undergraduate student. Several physician assistants provided an abundance of information and continual encouragement towards my educational goals. I also had the opportunity to see how patients improved their healthcare, listening to those patients' thoughts and seeing their satisfaction after treatment by a physician assistant. This encouraged me to join the field of serving and educating patients about healthcare as a physician assistant, and to eventually embrace the challenge of evaluating patients and developing a plan of care.

Third, during my undergraduate studies I spent time working with a variety of patients including children, athletes, working adults, and the elderly, and as a physician assistant, I can expect to continue to work with a diverse patient population. In addition, I enjoyed the camaraderie of working as part of a health care team; I believe this cultivated my interest in working in this environment, especially the opportunity to shadow several physician assistants.

Finally, throughout high school and college, I continued to challenge myself academically and personally. Immediately upon arriving at a college, I set out to make friends and join organizations. I served as a resident assistant for a year and a half; my college softball team voted me team captain my sophomore year. My professors have looked to me to provide leadership while working in the athletic training environment and class labs.

I have strong personal communication skills and am passionately motivated to continue increasing my health care knowledge and skills. I am confident that I will succeed as a physician assistant based on my previous experiences, successes, and personal attributes. More importantly, I look forward to serving and helping others achieve excellent healthcare.

Entering Your Academic History

If you are using the central application service for physician assistants, entering your academic history will probably be the most irritating and tedious part of the process. First, you must enter each institution you attended, followed by each class you took, the term it was taken in, and your grade. CASPA allows you to convert your grades so they are all formatted in the appropriate manner (this means you can enter in numeric and alphabetic grades you received). In order to enter in any of this information, you must have copies of your transcripts in front of you. Again, you do not want to enter any information incorrectly (even accidentally), so be sure to double-check everything.

In addition to entering all of your grades, you must also send CASPA an official copy of your transcript. You must print out the transcript request form (from the CASPA website in the section "Institutions Attended") and send it to **each** institution you attended. Some institutions charge a fee for your transcripts, and others do not. I would advise you to begin this process early so you can monitor, via the CASPA website, whether or not your transcripts have been received.

You should (of course) check to make sure the information below is current, but as this book's printing, you should send your official transcripts to the following address:

CASPA
Transcript Department
P.O. Box 9108
Watertown, MA 02471

Another part of CASPA's academic history portion is entering your standardized test information. According to the CASPA website, if you have not taken the GRE yet and your school requests it, you should designate that the GRE scores be sent to that particular school when you take the exam. However, if you have already taken the GRE, you can simply enter in your scores into the CASPA website; CASPA will then verify that information based on your social security number.

You should not request that your GRE scores be sent to CASPA—CASPA does not collect official GRE scores. Make sure that you have the scores sent to your selected schools if those schools require the GRE. If you are entering information about other standardized exams, such as the Medical College Admissions Test ("MCAT") or Test of English as a Foreign Language ("TOEFL"), please refer to the CASPA website—they have different requirements for these exams. For example, you must send a paper copy of your TOEFL scores to CASPA. You can also have these scores sent to the address listed above.

Letters of Recommendation

Obtaining letters of recommendation can range from fun to (more likely) excruciatingly painful. Here are my suggestions to make the process as painless as possible: first of all, you need to decide who to ask. Carefully consider who you will ask, as you want someone who will put you in the best light possible.

As of now, CASPA requires three letters of recommendation. Find out if the institutions you are applying to have any specific requirements about who the letters are written by. Some PA programs require the letters be written by physicians or physician assistants, while others have no requirements. You can have the person you choose either enter their letter electronically through a secure website, or send it via "paper" form—the ancient process where your recommender actually writes a letter and sends it to CASPA. It is wise to ask the person who will be writing the letter for you which way they would prefer to submit it, and help them if they need any assistance. Make it as easy as possible for your letter writers to submit their letters, and do not forget to follow up. You may need to reach out to your recommenders a number of times.

Understand at the onset that, at most institutions, letters of recommendation do not weigh extremely heavily in the scoring process when compared to grades and healthcare experience. But a letter of recommendation that is not favorable can still hurt you in the application process!

I know a person who applied to graduate school after attending a major university. In a very difficult chemistry class with nearly 400 students, she was one of 10 students to receive a 4.0 grade. She decided to ask the professor of that class to write her a recommendation letter because she thought that since she did so well in the class, he would think highly of her and write a great letter.

She was wrong! The professor did write a letter for her, but unfortunately the letter said very little that was positive about the student. The professor commended her for getting a good grade in his class, of course, but also said that he did not know her because the class was so large, and he had never worked with her one-on-one.

Learn from her mistake.   When deciding who to ask for a recommendation letter, choose someone that knows you very well—or can at least pick you out of a crowd.   The strongest letters of recommendation will come from professors, PAs, MDs, DOs, or nurses who know you well, who can verify that you have the drive to become a great physician assistant, and can opine that you will succeed in a rigorous academic environment.   If you shadowed a PA or physician, you may want to ask them for a letter.   You should also have a professor write you a letter of recommendation.   Make sure the professor you choose is someone who can comment on you favorably as a person, and not just state that you did well in his or her class.

Remember, it is your responsibility to get to know your professors, and to get to know a professional who will write you a strong letter of recommendation.   You simply must make this effort when you have the opportunity.   Keep addresses and contact information for each professional contact you meet.   You may want to become "friends" with these people on some of the social media sites in order to stay connected.   You never know when you will need to refer back to a contact you have met, so it is important to remain in touch.

When using CASPA for the electronic version of the letter of recommendation, you need to enter in all of the letter writer's personal information.   CASPA will then send that person an "electronic request" asking them to fill out your letter on their secured website.   You should follow-up with your letter writer to make sure they received the "electronic request" and to make sure they completed the letter of recommendation.   This is important because sometimes the electronic request from CASPA is accidentally deleted (or filtered into their spam e-mail) by the person you have asked to act as a personal reference.

One nice thing about the CASPA system is that you can check the status of your letters of recommendation and your transcripts to find out if they have been received, or if they are still pending.   Again, once you have asked people to write letters of recommendation for you, be it in electronic or paper form, it is your responsibility to monitor the status of your letters and to make sure those people you have asked complete them in a timely manner.

If you have asked someone to write a letter of recommendation for you, try to make the process easy for them by giving them written instructions as well as a current resume (so they know more about your background and future goals). And please, please send anyone who has written you a letter of recommendation a thank you note afterward.

As someone who has written nearly one hundred recommendation letters during my time teaching, I can assure you that writing recommendation letters is very time consuming. Thank those who wrote letters for you for the time they took out of their already busy schedules—and remember, you may need their help in the future so it is important to be professional.

Supplemental Applications

There should be no doubt by this point, but in case it is not yet clear: every school has a different way of doing things, and "one size" does not fit all. Some schools have you fill out the supplemental or secondary application (the two are interchangeable) at the same time you apply using the CASPA. Other schools send out supplemental applications at a later date, limiting recipients to qualified applicants.

In many cases, the supplemental application will ask you to fill out basic information, such as your personal contact information and your academic history—which you can easily copy from your CASPA application. At other schools, the supplemental application will instead ask you to answer essay questions. In order to make it through this next step, you will want to follow the directions on the secondary applications carefully.

While the CASPA website does specify whether or not you need to submit a supplemental application, also contact your specific school(s) to verify this information—it is not uncommon for a PA program to change its admission requirements from year to year, and CASPA is not perfect when updating every school's specific requirements.

Many schools provide information regarding supplemental or secondary applications on their website. Where applicable, I have included this information in the index of PA programs at the end of the book.

The goal of the supplemental applications is to allow the university to get a better sense of your depth of knowledge regarding healthcare in general, and specifically the PA profession. Additionally, the school uses this application as another step to help "weed out" applicants (typically those students who are not astute enough to complete the application within the requested time-frame).

The typical secondary application includes essay questions that the student must answer. If a student is not passionate about attending that particular school, it is possible that he or she will not take the time and energy required to complete the essay questions. So, by answering the questions and returning the secondary application before the due-date, you are placing yourself in a better position to move onto the next round of the admissions process.

If you receive a secondary application, the first thing you should do is read the directions very carefully. Second, you should make several copies of the application. Some applications require handwritten essays; so, if you find that you need to handwrite your answers, you will want to avoid using the original copy the first time you write it out. Just imagine—you have written out your essay on the original application, and realize, with ten words to go, that your essay, written lovingly in black ink, is so long it does not fit on the page. That has certainly happened to students before. Make sure it does not happen to you!

To start answering the questions, you should first do some research. Often, the questions are related to PA reimbursement, the role of the

PA in comparison to the NP or the physician, and some may even be a bit more personal—asking you to explain a personal story about your healthcare experience. Whatever the questions are, make sure you do the appropriate research. You can use whatever resources you need to—make sure you have read through this book in its entirety, talk to people, read articles on the internet, and look to PA organizations. I also encourage you to have several people read your essays to make sure they are grammatically correct and that they make sense.

When you have perfected your answers, practice writing them on the copies you made to confirm that they fit. Once each fits, write them on the original copies and make sure you write it in your best handwriting. I cannot tell you how many secondary applications I have seen where the handwriting is hardly even legible. When I am scoring essays and I see the applicant has not taken the time write legibly, while I try to remain unbiased, I am probably more inclined to score the essay poorly. I emphasize again, write the essays in your best handwriting.

Finally, pay attention to the deadline. Secondary applications are usually due within 2 weeks of receiving them. Make sure you send them out before the deadline so they arrive on-time. If you are concerned about the PA program not receiving the secondary application, you can always call the program, or send an e-mail to check. Back up your records by sending the application via certified US mail or an overnight service with package tracking.

When I applied to PA school, only one school required that its applicants complete secondary applications. Nowadays, secondary applications are used much more frequently. In order to give you an idea of what a secondary application may be like, I am listing some typical questions, followed by actual PA student answers. Again, please use these only as guides.

1. Explain how electronic medical records are changing the way healthcare providers practice medicine:

> As a registered dietitian, I have seen first-hand how the use of electronic medical records (EMR) has impacted patient care. My use of these systems has allowed me to retrieve patient

information, order specific diets for patients, and review pertinent lab data—all in one place. Utilizing electronic medical records has allowed me to work much more efficiently than I was when compared to paper medical charts. I have also found that I am able to review aspects of the patient charts easily, as I am no longer struggling to read illegible handwriting.

While there are many benefits to EMR, there are also some risks associated with using these systems. For example, there is a greater risk of violating patient privacy. As patient data is typically easier for clinicians to access, it is possible that clinicians may inappropriately use the system. Another risk of using EMR is the chance that the computer systems could lose data or "crash." While this is unlikely to occur, it is possible, and could be catastrophic if important patient data was lost, and/or medical errors occurred as a consequence. It is also important to recognize that there is a learning curve associated with using new technology, and lengthy training programs may temporarily impede from patient care.

As a physician assistant student, I look forward to learning how to use EMR responsibly. I know that having access to patient medical records is a privilege, and I plan on building on my past experiences to learn how I can use the systems to provide my patients with the most efficient and accurate care that I can.

2. *Explain why you want to become a PA:*

I have been passionate about becoming a PA since my freshman year of college. After being treated by a PA in the student health center, and being extremely impressed with her knowledge about my illness and the quality of care I received, I decided this was the perfect profession for me.

I love science and medicine, and I feel that working as a physician assistant will allow me to unite these two interests of mine throughout my career. Working as a physician assistant will also allow me to work in the healthcare field in any specialty—which is one of my favorite aspects of the profession. My father is a primary care physician and he has been extremely supportive of my decision to pursue a career as a PA. Working with him as a medical assistant in his private practice has allowed me to see how valuable mid-level providers can be when they work alongside physicians and other medical staff. I look forward to becoming a part of this integrated care system.

Over the past 4 years of college, I have completed science classes beyond the prerequisites in an effort to better prepare myself for PA school. I am excited to become a PA and look forward to all of the challenges that are ahead of me as I begin this difficult educational process.

3. *Explain an unforgettable healthcare experience you have had:*

As a nursing assistant, I was lucky enough to meet many great residents in the extended care facility I worked at. One patient in particular, George, was a favorite resident of mine. George was passionate about the game show, Jeopardy. Despite being elderly and relatively uneducated, he watched the show daily and knew many of the answers.

George was in the extended care facility because he had been diagnosed with stage 4 liver cancer. He, with his family's support, had opted to undergo chemotherapy, but no other forms of treatment (aside from pain management). His prognosis was grim from the day he entered our facility, but despite that, he was always very cheerful and kind.

Whenever I worked with George, we discussed some of the answers that had been on Jeopardy that particular day. Our last conversation was about technology. After watching the IBM computer, Watson, win an entire week on the game show, we talked about the many ways in which computers are changing the world. George encouraged me to become more comfortable with computers as he imagined that it would be an important part of my job in the future. Because I appreciated his opinion, and I agreed with him, I took a course this past semester in college to learn more about computers in medicine.

While I was deeply saddened when George passed away, I was also grateful that I had gotten the chance to meet him. My experience working with him helped reinforce the importance of getting to know each patient on a personal level.

4. Explain how you think the Patient Protection and Affordable Care Act of 2010 will impact physician assistants:

The Patient Protection and Affordable Care Act will play a significant role in how healthcare providers are able to treat patients. In many ways, patients will benefit from this legislation. For example, many patients who were unable to obtain health insurance will now be able to purchase a plan at a much lower cost. This will directly affect physician assistants as there will be a greater number of patients to care for. I think this will lead to an expansion in the number of PA training programs in the United States as there will be a greater demand for primary care providers.

I believe the increased number of patient visits will initially lead to difficulties for all providers as they will have to curtail the amount of time they are able to spend with each patient. As with current insurance plans and government programs, there will probably be limitations on the types of medications that can be prescribed and the types of treatments that patients will be able to receive due to restricted funding. Although there are a lot of potential difficulties that may occur with the implementation of the program, I think that providing every U.S. Citizen with a healthcare plan is a major victory and will ultimately make any hindrances seem minor in the end.

5. *Explain why you think more physician assistants are working in specialties:*

> There are several reasons that physician assistants are opting to work in specialty areas instead of primary care settings. First, many primary care clinics are supported by Medicare and Medicaid patients and oftentimes these patients pay lower premiums for healthcare. This makes it more difficult for physicians to afford physician assistants, despite the need for additional providers. Second, with the restricted number of hours that a resident physician may work, these hours are now being overturned to PAs working in hospital specialties. Third, with the increased desire to specialize on the part of physicians, PAs are following their lead and are working directly with them. Lastly, physician assistants may choose to work in specialty because some areas of medicine provide higher salaries than others. Despite all of the reasons that physician assistants may choose to work in specialty areas, there is still a significant need for PAs to work in primary care settings.

Don't Forget: A Few Things to Remember about CASPA

Using the CASPA system costs money. And, unfortunately, the more schools you apply to, the more money it costs. As of now, the current cost for CASPA starts at $135 for one school and adds an additional $30-$40 for each additional school you apply to. So, if you apply to four schools through CASPA, it will likely cost you over $200. Budget for this amount from the beginning, but understand that you will not pay the CASPA fee until you actually click "submit" and send all of your information to CASPA.

Remember to send these items via U.S. Mail to CASPA:

- Letters of Recommendation—either electronically or in paper form
- Transcripts—make sure you order and send official copies

If you have problems with CASPA, do not hesitate to call them. I spoke with them when I had questions during my application, and they were quite helpful. As of now, you can reach CASPA at:

Telephone: 617-612-2080
E-Mail: CaspaInfo@caspaonline.org

The CASPA Checklist

This checklist/chart should help you organize the materials you will need to successfully complete the CASPA process, and actually completing this chart will help you determine whether or not you are ready to "E-submit" your CASPA application. Once you have completed all of the items on the checklist, you should feel confident that you are ready to send your application on for admissions review.

Have I completed the following?	YES
Ordered my Transcripts	
Selected three people to write Letters of Recommendation and sent those people the CASPA Information **1.** **2.** **3.**	
Sent in my Supplemental Applications **(If your schools require these)**	
Carefully entered my GRE Information **(If required to)**	
Carefully entered my Contact Information	
Carefully entered my Personal Data	
Carefully entered my Additional Information	
Carefully entered my Health Related Training	
Read my Personal Statement out loud	
Had friends and family read and review my Personal Statement	
Carefully Spell-Checked and Grammar-Checked my Personal Statement	
Carefully entered my Narrative or Personal Statement	
Carefully entered my Work and Volunteer Experience	
Carefully entered my Institutions Attended	
Carefully entered my Coursework	
Carefully entered the Programs I want CASPA to send my Information to	
Double Checked all of the Above!	

The Interview Process

If you have received an interview, congratulations! Now that you have the opportunity to show the school who you are in person, you should make the most of it. Of course, that opportunity may be unique depending on the location—interviews can be quite different from school to school. Some schools interview as many as 50 students, all on one day; others may only interview a few students at one time. Some interviews will last the entire day and others may be finished in 30 minutes. This means one thing: be prepared for anything.

The typical interview day begins with a "welcome" session where potential students are introduced to some of the faculty members, and is often followed by a tour of the school and some of the classrooms. Finally, students are interviewed by a few different members of the faculty and, in some cases, by students currently enrolled in the program.

During some interviews students may be asked to participate in a quick writing test. Be prepared: do not party late the night before, since schools use this test to assess your ability to think and write clearly in a short amount of time. If you are given a test, do your best to think quickly and answer to the best of your abilities.

Remember to write legibly on the test as educators do look at penmanship. Most of the time, the questions on these tests are straightforward and ask general questions about the profession or your opinion about an issue within the profession. If you are reading this book, you will be well-prepared to answer these questions, as we will cover most of the important topics about the profession throughout the book.

In order to fully prepare for the interview, you need to do some research first. You will need to learn about the PA program you are interviewing at, as well as more about the profession in general. Create a "cheat-sheet" for yourself by developing a document that contains some of the key information about the school you are interviewing at. You can do this by reviewing the PA program's website.

You should include the following in your "cheat-sheet":

- The focus of the training program (primary care, surgery, etc.)
- The number of students in each class
- Some of the names of the professors and their areas of expertise (especially if you find out beforehand that they are attending)
- At least two reasons why you want to specifically attend this PA program (you can include more if you have them)
- At least two reasons why you think the school should select you to be in the class (you can include more if you have them)

Print out this document with information about your school, and bring it with you for reference. Review the document while you are waiting to be interviewed.

You will also need to practice answering some sample interview questions out loud. Have a family member or friend ask you practice questions so you can get used to answering them. By answering the questions out loud, you may realize that you do not really know what you are talking about. I suggest you research the following questions. You may or may not be asked these questions, but it never hurts to be prepared.

Topics you should be comfortable talking about should include:

- The role of the PA in healthcare
- The difference between PAs, NPs, and MDs or DOs
- How PAs are reimbursed
- Different practice settings PAs can practice in
- Why you want to be a PA
- Why the PA program should choose you
- How you will deal with the stress of the program
- What type of work you want to do as a PA (Family practice, plastic surgery, etc.)
- Why you are interested in this specific PA program
- How you are unique from other PA candidates the school is interviewing
- What are your own strengths and weaknesses?

- What are your hobbies?
- Do you work well with others, or do you prefer to work by yourself?
- How does your family feel about you going to PA school?
- What will you do if you are not accepted to PA school?
- What do you imagine PA school will be like?
- What do you imagine PA practice will be like?

Some programs like to throw in random questions to see how you will respond. If you are asked a silly question, such as, "If you were an animal, what animal would you choose to be?" just answer the question as creatively and quickly as you can. Do not worry—they simply want to see if you can think on your feet.

You may also get asked questions that relate to current trends in healthcare or scenarios that you might find yourself in as a PA. It is hard to prepare for these types of broad questions, but I recommend doing some research to make sure you have a basic understanding of the current laws related to PA reimbursement, and Medicare/Medicaid. (You can learn more about these topics in this book).

As for health scenarios, I can give you an example:

> You are the PA working in the Emergency Room and you are evaluating a 14-year-old girl who presented with abdominal pain. After examining her, your nurse informs you that the urine sample you ordered earlier shows a very high level of Beta hCG indicating that your patient is likely pregnant. What do you do?

Questions like these are difficult to answer, and if you are given one similar to this, just try to answer it the best you can. If you do not understand something, it is ok for you to say, "I don't know," or, "I am not sure." Remember, you are not a PA yet, so you should not be expected to know everything that a PA would know already.

By giving you questions like these, interviewers are just trying to assess your ability to think critically and to give sound, reasonable answers. If you are unsure of the answer they are looking for, explain that under these circumstances, you would look up the answer in order to make sure you could correctly diagnose and treat the patient.

You may also be asked to explain basic science concepts. I have met PA educators who like to quiz students on areas of science that pre-PA students should be familiar with. For example, you may be asked to describe what a red blood cell is. If asked such a question, it is likely you will be thrown off a bit. And, quite honestly, the PA educator expects this. However, they are interested in finding out if you can recall information on the spot.

If you have no idea what the answer is, the best way to deal with the situation is to say what little you do know and then confidently inform the interviewer that you will look up the answer as soon as you leave the room (and, do it!). You want to demonstrate a desire to continue learning and the ability to complete a task efficiently when it is assigned.

Below is an example of how one might respond if asked a question he or she does not know the answer to.

- Question: What can you tell me about the Citric Acid Cycle is and its importance?

- Acceptable answers:

  - The Citric Acid Cycle (or Krebs Cycle) is a series of reactions which is important for all living cells as it leads to the creation of energy. (You could provide more details if you desired, but this would be an acceptable answer).

  - I remember learning about the Citric Acid Cycle in biology; however, at the moment I am very nervous and am having trouble recalling the specific details. I know that the cycle is important for energy production, but beyond that I would need to refer to a book to refresh myself—which, I will do as soon as I leave this room.

During the interview, there is usually an opportunity to ask your own questions. Most of the time, you will (or should) have had most of your questions answered by this point; however, if there are any items you still are curious about, this is your opportunity to ask. But be sure to ask your question carefully. You do not want to appear as though you have not done your research about the program, or as though you were not paying attention to what the interviewer has already told you.

A good way to ask a question may be to say, "I have reviewed the website and have spoken to several faculty members, so most of my questions have already been answered. However, I was wondering if you could tell me a little bit more about what I can expect regarding the next step in the application process. Will I be required to participate in another interview?" Whichever way you decide to ask your question, just be sure that you are polite and confident—without appearing pushy. And while a question or two are fine, do not ask *too* many questions—the fine line is appearing interested without appearing though you did not take the time to learn about the program before-hand.

Here are some questions you may wish to consider asking (if they were not already answered):

- Why should I choose your program?
- What is a typical day like during the didactic portion?
- What is a typical day like during the clinical portion?
- Are there any special programs for which this PA school is noted?
- How well do your students typically do on the PANCE exam?
- Has this PA school ever been on probation or had its accreditation revoked?
- How are students evaluated academically? (GPA, Pass/Fail, etc.)
- Is there a mechanism in place for students to evaluate their professors and attending physicians?
- Are there any scholarships within the program I can apply for?
- What kind of academic and personal counseling opportunities are available to students?

- Are there computer facilities available to students?
- Are computers or electronic medical programs integrated into the curriculum or learning activities?
- Is there a specific type of computer or electronic device I will be required to have?
- What type of learning modalities does the program use? (Problem-based learning, lecture, hands-on, etc.)
- Before I begin the program, are there any additional courses or work experiences I should try to take advantage of?
- How long does it take for most graduates of your program to find jobs?
- What type of preparation do you provide your students with before taking the PANCE exam?
- Is a car necessary for clinical rotations? If so, are parking passes provided?
- Are students involved in community service?
- Are there any opportunities for rotations abroad?
- Does the school have a cadaver lab? If not, how is anatomy taught?
- Will I be taking classes with other medical students or physical therapy students, or is the program completely separate?

Take notes! If you attend a number of student interviews, at the end, you may not be able to differentiate between schools. Good note-taking will help remind you of each school's strengths and weaknesses.

Keep in mind that a strong interview may win over faculty members, even if your record includes weaker academic achievements. But because faculty members interview so many applicants, it is easy to distinguish those students who are prepared from who are not. If you are a young applicant, it is likely that you have not had much experience interviewing in the past, and this is oftentimes quite obvious. Even though you may not have had much experience with professional interviewing, you can improve your chances of success by practicing beforehand. I cannot emphasize the importance of this enough!

I recall a day of conducting interviews for physician assistant admissions when two particular students stood out to me. Applicant "A" was extremely strong on paper. And after reading through the entirety of her application before beginning the interview, I felt that I would probably recommend offering her a spot to our admissions committee solely based on her educational background and healthcare experience. Here, Applicant "A" is aptly named—she had a very high grade point average, and also had over 2,000 hours of patient care experience through her work as a nursing assistant.

However, upon meeting Applicant "A" in person, I was instantly disappointed. She was shy and awkward, and did not demonstrate one iota of the confidence I feel PA students need to make it through the program. To this day, I do not know if Applicant "A" believed that being "sweet" during her interview would be enough to get her into PA school when combined with her admittedly impressive credentials, but it did not work for me. Based on further conversations with colleagues, I do not believe that it wins over other interviewers either. Although she had dressed the part and certainly had a terrific background, she lacked confidence and interviewed poorly. Applicant "A" had not prepared for the interview in a manner that permitted me to view her as a viable candidate.

I ended up suggesting that we put Applicant "A" on the wait-list because she did so poorly in the interview. Her interview told me that she would not be a successful student in our program at this time. PA work requires taking initiative and on-the-spot critical thinking, are characteristics that are necessary in order to appropriately treat complex medical or surgical patients. Sadly, the interview with Applicant "A" demonstrated neither.

Applicant "B" was memorable in a different fashion—confident, eager, and intelligent, Applicant "B" took active control of her interview. She had prepared and it was evident.

Applicant "B" was able to answer my questions with a smile and with enthusiasm—almost as if she was excited that I had asked her that particular question. She provided unique anecdotes to familiar ques- tions—which, I really liked. For example, when I asked her if she had ever been involved in something unethical, she told me about a story about a fellow paramedic who had denied having a medical illness in order to continue working. Applicant "B" said the situation became uncomfortable for her because she saw the illness affect her colleague's clinical judgment on one occasion. Although she felt horrible doing it, she had to tell her supervisor what had happened. Her coworker was put on medical leave until the issue was resolved, and was not happy about it. She said that she felt patient care was more important than friendship at work—which is a lesson that is important to learn if you want to be a successful physician assistant.

When I asked Applicant "B" to tell me more about her personal weaknesses, she mentioned that she often forgets people's first names. She mentioned that she did not realize this was a problem until she was working as a paramedic and she could not remember her patient's names without constantly referring to their charts. She explained that she has been working on the problem by trying to use the person's name multiple times within the first few minutes of meeting them.

(As an aside, the answers I commonly hear to the "personal weakness question" are, "I have perfectionist characteristics;" "I over-analyze things;" "I have difficulties with time management;" and "I find myself taking on too much responsibility." Your interviewers have heard these all before. If you want to stand out, don't be "cute," and stay away from these trite answers).

As I was reviewing the application for Applicant "B," I noticed that her grade point average was a little bit lower than some of the others I had interviewed. However, she was more passionate about becoming a PA than others I had interviewed, and I really appreciated that. For that reason, I recommended that we accept this student. And, for the record, she did matriculate in the program, and ended up being one of the leaders in the class.

Another tip is a simple one: when you are interviewing for a position in a PA program, be polite and courteous to everyone on campus—you never know who you might run into! Bad behavior can ruin your chances of acceptance. Imagine you have just completed your interview, and you decide to make a stop in the bathroom before leaving campus. Your mom calls you while you are in the restroom and asks you how the interview went. You tell her that you survived, but that you did not really like that they mentioned some of the students might have to do some rotations at an off-site community hospital a few hours away from campus. You tell your mother that you told them what they wanted to hear, but that you would never actually allow yourself to do a rotation in that particular place because it is too far away and too small for you to learn anything useful.

What you did not realize was that the person washing her hands in the bathroom while you were chatting was one of the PA faculty members that you did not meet. You also did not realize that this faculty member immediately conveyed what she heard in the bathroom to the program director. However, you are very aware that *something* happened when four weeks later you receive a letter informing you that you were not accepted into the program. Can you guess how much "hypothetical" there is in the above anecdote?

Professionalism is important, especially if you want to attend physician assistant school and work in this field. This is a profession, not a job, and character expectations come with the title. Character, in turn, represents those actions you take when you think no one else is looking (or can hear you in the restroom). It is important to be kind to everyone you meet or talk to throughout the application process for a particular program. If you are inadvertently (or intentionally) rude, impolite, or simply oblivious when interacting with someone, this may significantly impact your ability to gain acceptance into a program.

And, it should go without saying, the same holds true for your "virtual self"—the same exact story could hold true if the dialog had occurred on an open Facebook profile or like service. Before I get off my soapbox, I want to conclude with the following: if you want to be successful in life, and certainly in this profession, you will have to learn to be polite and courteous to everyone in your professional life—and, to be safe, you may as well extend that courtesy to everyone period.

There are, of course, some other interview tips you should have, and I have included this list to present some general ideas about your presentations:

- You should dress to impress. Whether you are male or female, you should definitely wear a suit. I have seen people show up at interviews wearing khaki pants and a polo shirt and they look uncomfortable and completely out of place. Do not let that happen to you! Dress as professionally as possible and groom yourself appropriately. Remember, to a large degree you are selling yourself, so you want to look your best.
- Bring a notepad and pen. Ask if you can take notes, and then jot down ideas while still maintaining eye contact. This will show you are interested in what the school representatives have to say.
- Do not chew gum! Instead, for hygiene purposes, keep some breath mints in your pocket.
- Look the interviewer in the eye. Try to concentrate on what they are saying and demonstrate that you are interested in what they have to say.
- Shake hands at the beginning of the interview when you introduce yourself. Pay attention to the interviewer's name. After the interview, thank them for their time by using their name (if you need to, jot it down on your notepad!).
- Smile during the interview and appear enthusiastic about the program.
- Do not act inappropriately or immature. Enough said.
- Arrive on-time. In fact, commit to arriving 15-20 minutes early! If you are traveling long distances to get there, make arrangements to be early. Use a map program to provide clear directions. The last thing you want to do is show up late, demonstrating that you do not appreciate their time.
- If you are very nervous, it is ok to tell the interviewer that. If you think your anxiety will seriously affect how you interview, it is ok to tell the interviewer, "I'm feeling a little bit nervous and excited today." While the interviewer may or may not take this into account, at least you have covered your bases.
- As the interview ends, ask for contact information or a business card from each person. Then, send a **handwritten** thank you

card to those people you met with and interviewed with, letting them know were grateful to have the opportunity to meet with them in person.

- If you do not have additional time constraints, visit the city and the neighborhood either the day before or the day after the interview. You are already there, so make the most of your trip. You might not get another chance, because of time or financial limitations, to revisit all of the locations again.
- Do yourself a favor and read the book, "How to Ace the Physician Assistant Interview" by Andrew J. Rodican. If you have any anxiety, reading the book is worth the time and money.

The bottom line: this may be your only opportunity to go to the school, meet the faculty, and see the facilities before you make a school decision. Make the most of this opportunity! It is your job to promote yourself and to explain why they should choose you, and not Jim or Jane Doe who happen to look exactly like you do (on paper). Practice answering questions beforehand, smile, and finally **remember to relax.**

The Waiting Game

The PA application process can be lengthy, time-consuming, expensive, and emotionally exhausting. However, like all things in life, the end will arrive at some point. And, there is little mystery in the process—every application ends in one of three ways: acceptance, wait-listing, or rejection.

Acceptance

If you are accepted to a PA program, congratulations! You should be incredibly proud of yourself. Luckily, you are finished with the stresses specifically associated with the application process.

If you have been accepted to a program you plan to attend, make your timely deposit payment your first priority, in order to reserve your spot in the program as soon as possible. As happened with one of my friends, it would be awful to receive an acceptance but neglect to pay the deposit necessary to secure your place in the program. As you did before, send your deposit check with a return receipt requested.

If you have been accepted to one PA program, but are still waiting to hear back from your first choice school, you are in a difficult position. In this case, you may have to pay the deposit to guarantee your spot in at least one program, or risk not having a spot at any PA program. Unfortunately, this happened to me. I had to pay the $500 deposit to hold my spot in the first PA program I was accepted to, while waiting to find out if I had gotten into my first choice. The idea of a school making you pay this fee is frustrating, but they need to know quickly whether or not you are going to matriculate into their program (but, to clarify, not all PA programs will make you pay a deposit to hold your spot).

Most PA programs have many students waiting to get in—so if you decide to relinquish your spot, it is very likely that the school will give it away to another student. If you do matriculate into a PA program, the deposit you pay goes towards your tuition. However, if you have paid the fee and do not end up attending the PA program, the fee will not be refunded. Make sure you budget for this potential "hidden" cost. And, this cost can be a lot—some schools require a deposit of more than $1,000.

It is also important to realize that each school should provide you with some type of "Technical Standards" form when you accept a position in their program. This form will contain information about the essential qualities and abilities necessary for you to be a successful student in their particular PA program. You must review these standards careful-ly, as you will want to confirm that you can appropriately comply with them before committing to your spot.

Dealing with the Wait-List

If you have been wait-listed, take a deep breath, but do not worry. You have joined a long and distinguished group of students. As you may know from college, wait-listing is what PA schools do when they have offered most of their spots to applicants, but are still waiting to find out if those applicants will matriculate into the program. While being wait-listed is disappointing, it does mean that you are still being considered for a spot. I have known several students who have matriculated into the PA program of their choice after being put on the wait-list.

If you have been wait-listed, you have not relinquished all control—and there is still more you can do. Send a letter to the PA program demonstrating your continued desire to be a part of their program and explain why you believe you are a good fit. You should mention any activities you are currently participating in (e.g. volunteering or taking a biology course) that may further demonstrate your commitment to the profession. Take this opportunity to augment your application with new, pertinent information that may not have been available when you first applied.

You may also want to consider sending an additional letter of recommendation. Not all programs will actually use these items to help make their decision as to whether or not you gain admission, but it will not hurt to try, and these actions will only potentially benefit you.

If you have been wait-listed, and have been accepted at another PA program, maybe you should consider releasing your spot on the wait-list. If you think you will be just as happy going to PA school somewhere that has already accepted you, then go there. Additionally, this will free up a spot for someone else who is likely on that school's wait-list. Unless you have a great reason to see it through, I would encourage you to avoid the additional stress of waiting to hear back from the school that wait-listed you. My advice is to pay the deposit where you have been accepted, and move on with your life. You should be happy you are going to PA school and do not have to worry about the application process anymore!

Be aware that students who are on the wait-list may not receive an offer of acceptance until very close to the beginning of the program. I have known students who were not informed of their PA school acceptance until just a few days before the program was set to begin. This can be very challenging as a student for several reasons. It is likely that you will have to move closer to the school before beginning a program, which can be difficult to do with only a few days notice. Additionally, you may not have made arrangements with your employer to leave on such short notice—leaving a job without properly notification is unprofessional and might leave lasting, unpleasant feelings between you and your employer (which would be unfortunate if your employer was a hospital or physician you may wish to work for in the future).

Keep in mind that many students who are accepted to PA programs begin communicating with one another months before the programs actually begin, so some students will have already found roommates and developed friendships before they actually set foot on campus for school.

If you are admitted at the last minute, you may miss out on this bonding and feel a little left out at first. However, if you know you want to be in the program, and you are willing to accept the added stress of matriculating at the last minute, then you should definitely proceed with admission—PA school is long, and there is plenty of time to catch up socially. If you have concerns about making all of the necessary changes on such short notice, you may want to ask the program if there is any possibility of deferring your acceptance until the next academic year so that you can adequately prepare. Depending on the school, deferment may or may not be an option.

While you are waiting to find out if you have been accepted, I would encourage you to continue to pursue activities that will make you a stronger applicant. Remember, it is a real possibility that you may not receive an acceptance this year and that you may have to reapply. By moving forward with your educational goals throughout the process, you can gain more healthcare experience or take additional coursework, thus making yourself a stronger applicant in the future.

Dealing with Rejection

If you have been rejected, it is not the end of the world (even though it may feel like it). And if you have never experienced rejection like this before, getting through this may be even more difficult because it was unexpected and your coping skills might be undeveloped. (Remember that support system I mentioned before when you were trying to decide whether you should go to PA school, well now is the time to rely on them a bit). It is alright to take a few days to experience the sadness associated with a failed plan.   Do your best to let go of the disappointment, and then move on.   Remember, that in life, things do not always go according to plan; this holds true in patient care as well—even the best physician assistants have patients that fail medical treatments despite all of their efforts.

You may be wondering, what do I do now?   Well, you have a few different options.   First of all, you should rethink the decision as to whether or not you really want to be a PA.   Think this through carefully.   Do you really want to go through the application process again?   As a personal decision, is it worth it to you?   If you choose to abandon the PA profession, I wish you well in whatever career endeavors you pursue.   However, if you decide you still want to become a PA, you will have to go through this entire process again. Take a moment to reflect, and take a deep breath, but then re-motivate yourself.

First, I suggest you call the schools that did not accept you and ask them specifically why you did not get in.   Be professional, not confrontational.   Find out what the reason was.   Was your GPA too low?   Did they think you needed more healthcare experience?   Did you interview poorly?   Whatever it is, you need to find out so that you can work on that specifically in anticipation for the next round of applications.

Focus on making yourself a stronger applicant this second (or third, or fourth) time around.   You have already been through the process, so you have a terrific idea of what you can expect.   Carefully go through this book and see if there was anything you missed.   Consider applying to different PA programs than you did initially.   Since you will have some extra time, try to get more healthcare experience.   Contact the PA you shadowed before and ask if you can shadow him or her again.

Take a certification course—possibly a nursing assistant course or an EMT course.   Join a PA organization and attend a conference where you can network with PAs and educators from different locations. Contact PA organizations and ask if they have any mentoring programs or if anyone might be willing to review your materials before you apply again.

Whatever you do, work on improving your application. You need to show the schools you are applying to that you really want to be a PA, and that you will do whatever it takes to become one. You may even want to talk about your initial rejection in your personal statement. If being rejected from PA school influenced you to want to try even harder to get in, then you may want to share that experience with the programs you are applying to. PA programs will want to know what you have done to make yourself a stronger applicant if you were rejected once before.

Just remember that whatever happens, whether you are accepted or rejected, you will still be the same person that you were before. These may sound like empty platitudes, but no matter what the outcome is, you will still have the same drive and the same desire to help people, and even if being a PA was not meant for you, there are plenty of other great careers you can pursue.

Part V: Surviving PA School

Paying for PA School

Most PA students (and their families) cannot afford to pay the high cost of tuition up front; however, there are several options for students who will need assistance. We will discuss a number of those options in this chapter.

Loans

The first option is student loans. There are different types of loans, and some are clearly preferable to others. A federal loan may the best type of student loan available, because the interest rate is almost always lower than private loans. The current fixed interest rate (as of 2011) on most federal loans for graduate students is 6.8%.[37] There are two different types of federal loans: subsidized and unsubsidized. Subsidized loans are based on financial need, and there is no interest charged or accumulated while you are in school. Unsubsidized loans are not based on financial need and do accumulate interest while you are in school. Therefore subsidized loans have the added benefit of remaining interest-free until you must begin repayment. Unfortunately, you are currently limited to $20,500 in federal loans per year for tuition costs (and no more than $8,500 of that amount can be subsidized). As discussed before, this is unlikely to cover all of your financial needs.[38]

Repayment with student loans is quite flexible, and currently there are four different plans you can choose: the standard plan, the extended plan, the graduated plan, and the income-based plan.[39] For repayment, the loans have a 6 month grace period so you do not actually have to make your first payment until you have been out of school for 6

---

[37] Federal Student Aid: Calculators and Interest Rates. Available online at: http://www.direct.ed.gov/calc.html. Accessed on August 22, 2011.
[38] The SmartStudent Guide to Financial Aid: Student Loans. Available online at: http://www.finaid.org/loans/studentloan.phtml. Accessed on August 22, 2011.
[39] Federal Student Aid: Repayment Plans. Available online at: http://www.direct.ed.gov/RepayCalc/dlindex2.html. Accessed on August 22, 2011.

months. If you are interested in applying for federal loans, you will need to fill out the same Free Application for Federal Student Aid ("FAFSA") form you may have used as an undergraduate student, which you can get from your school's financial aid office.

To find out more about federal student loans, you should check out the Government's website at:
http://www.ed.gov/offices/OSFAP/DirectLoan/student.html.

In addition to federal student loans, most physician assistant students will also need to take out private loans in order to cover the cost of living and any additional tuition costs. There are several different companies who provide students with private loans. Each school has arrangements with different lenders, so you may or may not have a choice in the matter. Private loans typically have higher interest rates than federal loans. The interesting thing about private loans is that you will receive the loan in the form of a personal check, and you have the responsibility to make sure it goes to the right places (rent, food, excess tuition, transportation, etc.). **Be careful!** Usually, you must make this money last for 8-12 months before you receive another check.

If you are wise, you will be thoughtful about budgeting beforehand and will only take out the amount of money (from private loans) that you will actually need. This will keep you from borrowing any "extra" money. Remember, whatever you take out, you will have to pay back with interest. Although extra money can make life a little easier while you are in PA school, it is very difficult to pay back high interest rate loans. Private loans typically have different repayment plans than federal loans. I was surprised to find out that my private loan only had one repayment option. **Make sure you have carefully reviewed your loan materials before you commit—you need to know what you are signing up for when it comes to student loans.**

Once you have been accepted to a PA program, you will be given information regarding financial aid through your PA program. In addition, the PA program should have a financial aid advisor who can help determine which payment plan is right for you.

Scholarships

Unlike undergrad, where students may attend on full-scholarship, the typical PA student gets little to nothing when it comes to tuition assistance from his or her PA program. That being said, there are some exceptions to this, and there are scholarships that you can apply for.

First, find out if your university offers any specific scholarships for PA students. One of the universities I worked for offered a partial tuition scholarship for graduate health students. Those students awarded the scholarship received monies from the university that covered nearly half of their tuition expenses. While these scholarships are highly competitive, they are worth applying to if available.

If you want to go to PA school for free, your best bet is the National Health Service Corps ("NHSC"). Students selected as NHSC scholars receive full tuition and fee reimbursement, in addition to a monthly stipend throughout their education. But there is a catch: a NHSC student must provide two years of service in a primary care setting that is recognized by the program as medically underserved. Before applying to this program, take a look at the list of potentially "medically underserved" areas online. Oftentimes the locations you may be assigned to are quite rural, and you will want to take this into consideration when deciding whether or not this program is appealing to you.

If you plan to participate in the NHSC program, you should apply as soon as possible. Applications are typically due in the spring, and recipients are notified of their status in the Fall of that year. Be forewarned, the program is very competitive. According to their website, the NHSC receives seven applications for each spot. As of now, the current website can be accessed at: http://nhsc.bhpr.hrsa.gov /scholarship/.

The AAPA supplies several PA students with scholarships through their Physician Assistant Foundation. As of now, the website can be accessed at: http://www.aapa.org/pa-foundation/scholarships-and-grants. The application process may vary from year to year, but it generally requires a few essays as well as a letter of recommendation.

The PA Foundation scholarships are competitive, but, if you can get assistance it will, of course, be worth it.

Another option may to join the United States military. Joining the military when you begin PA school can provide many benefits. Each service branch has different programs, but generally students make a 2-3 year commitment to serve in the military after the completion of PA school in order to receive full tuition assistance as well as a monthly stipend during PA school. A friend of mine is currently serving time in the United States Air Force as a physician assistant, and he has been very happy with his decision to pursue this path. Make sure you find out all of the details before making the commitment though—you will want to be fully informed of all the post-education service obligations before you join.

For those potential applicants currently in the military, the Interservice Physician Assistant Program ("IPAP") is a viable option. While highly competitive, the program requires no tuition fees for selected students. Following completion of this two year program, students are awarded a master's degree and are eligible to take the national certification exam for PAs. The program is located in Fort Sam Houston, Texas, and graduates receive a commission as a First Lieutenant in the Army Medical Specialist Corps, with a post-education service commitment. Anyone serving in the military, regardless of their service, can apply for an active duty Army training seat to become eligible to participate in the IPAP program.

I have also known students who were "sponsored" by a hospital to attend physician assistant school. These students worked at the hospital before attending PA school and signed a contract with the hospital agreeing to return to work for the institution following the successful completion of their physician assistant training. The hospital then paid the student's tuition during PA school. Not many hospitals offer this option; however, if you are currently employed by a hospital (or by a private physician with whom you get along with very well), you should certainly explore the possibility of such an agreement.

There are several other PA organizations that offer scholarships as well; here are just a few:

- American Association of Surgical Physician Assistants (http://www.aaspa.com/)
- Association of Physician Assistants in Cardiovascular Surgery (http://www.apacvs.org/)
- Physician Assistants in Orthopaedic Surgery (http://www.paos.org/)
- Society of Emergency Medicine Physician Assistants (http://www.sempa.org/)
- Association of Family Practice Physician Assistants (http://www.afppa.org/)
- Society for Physician Assistants in Pediatrics (http://www.spaponline.org/)
- Society of Physician Assistants in Otorhinolaryngology / Head & Neck. Surgery (http://www.entpa.org/)

Additionally, several state PA organizations offer scholarships to student members. Check with your state PA organizations to see if they offer any scholarships you can apply for.

Finally, check back in with your financial aid counselor at your PA program. He or she may know of some scholarships within the program that you can apply for.

Budgeting 101

Not only is being in PA school mentally and physically taxing, it is also financially taxing! When you are a PA student, you must learn to live on a budget. Most PA students will be living on loan money throughout the duration of the program, and may be living in a locale that is more expensive than they are used to. Regardless, the average PA student must commit to living frugally.

While easier said than done, I suggest you create a budget for yourself and stick to it. You do not want to run out of money halfway through the school year and have to apply for more private loan aid. Stick with your budget and live below your means. Pay for the essentials, such as food and transportation, but stay away from the non-essentials such as clothing and entertainment. During your clinical period, you will be likely live in hospital-provided scrubs anyway. I know it is tough! Trust me, I have been there, but living like a student for a few years will benefit you in the long run. Besides, your peer group of fellow students will be doing the same thing.

To help you, I have included a budget checklist. Take the time to fill it out now, and revisit it as you prepare to begin school. A little planning at this stage of the process can save you thousands of dollars in future costs and interest payments.

In addition to mapping out your budget using a checklist like the one provided, I would also recommend that you utilize resources online to help you plan. One excellent resource for estimating how much PA school will cost is available at the Physician Assistant ED website (http://www.physicianassistanted.com). The website has a "True Cost to Attend Calculator" that allows you to compare the different costs of various PA programs.

The Budget Checklist

Anticipated Costs	Year One	Year Two	Year Three?
Tuition			
Health Insurance			
Housing			
Food			
Transportation			
Books			
Medical Equipment			

TOTAL COSTS

I apologize if this seems too straightforward to bother with an explanation, but to estimate your total costs above, please add up the sums of Years One through Three—this will give you the approximate costs for expenses that are directly school-related. This is a general baseline for your expense—you must also include all of the extra expenses listed on the next page.

After you have worked through the entire worksheet, you will have a much better idea of what you should expect to spend on PA school. This will also arm you with information you can use when distinguishing between comparable PA schools on the basis of cost.

"Other" Fees	Year One	Year Two	Year Three?
Computer / PDA			
Certifications (BCLS, ACLS, PALS)			
Student Malpractice Insurance			
Student Disability Insurance			
Gym Membership			
TV / Cable / Phone			
Gas / Car Insurance / Maintenance			
Laboratory Fee(s)			
University Activity Fee(s)			
Student Health Fee(s)			
Graduation Fee			
PANCE (exam-related fees and study materials)			
Family Expenses (if you are married or are a parent)			
Travel Expenses (if you are attending a program far away from home)			
Miscellaneous			

TOTAL COSTS _____

As you can see, the costs add up very quickly. By creating a budget and examining your finances before you begin PA school, you are already taking steps to prevent accumulating more debt than you can afford.

The Didactic Phase "Pearls"

Most physician assistant programs are about 26 months in length and are divided into two separate parts: the didactic portion and the clinical portion. The two parts are quite different in terms of what and how you will be learning.

The didactic portion of any PA school is the most mentally challenging aspect of the program. In fact, this is the part of the program that many students fail to complete. Most programs are set up so that students have class all day long, from 8 a.m. until 6 or 7 p.m., commonly with several exams per week. This means that, after a long day in the classroom or laboratory, you must study for several hours each night in order to try to retain the information. It can be overwhelming. The expectations for you as a PA student are extremely high, and in order to survive the program, you have to find a way to make school your number one priority.

Pay Attention in Class

In PA school, students are typically presented with large volumes of information in lecture format. I know it is easy to "zone out" during lectures, to play on your computer, or to send text messages to your friends. However, it is your responsibility to learn all of the core principles of medicine during this short didactic period before beginning clinical rotations.

Paying attention in class can make learning these principles much easier. Try to think of your brain as a sponge, with its purpose to absorb as much of the information as it possibly can. You will, inevitably, forget information that you have learned along the way, but if you make an effort to pay attention in class and soak up as much as you can, you will have an easier time recalling information when you actually need it.

It is easy to lose interest during a lecture, but it is important to find ways to keep engaged. Some students find they focus much better if they turn all of their technology off during class (no computer, or mobile devices)—thus, reducing their likelihood of being distracted. Other students find they need to take notes during class—either electronically or by hand—in order to pay attention.

You may find that reviewing the lecture notes briefly before class may highlight areas of the presentation that might be of particular interest to you. Do your best to find a way to stay energized during class—and experiment with different methods until you find what works for you. I have a few suggestions to help get you started: stay hydrated, get up and move around during breaks (fresh air can be extremely helpful), chew gum, use caffeine responsibly, get to know your professors so that you feel comfortable discussing topics of interest to you in class, and do not forget to eat small healthy snacks throughout the day.

Find an Effective Way to Study

Each student learns material differently, and you may find that you have to study more (or less) than some of your classmates. You may also find that the methods you used to study in undergrad are not effective for you anymore. I encourage you to utilize multiple methods as a combination can all help reinforce your knowledge of material.

Some people study well in groups. If you believe you are one of these people, form a study group with some of your classmates. Each of you can take on certain topics and teach them to the other members of the group. Or, each of you can type up summaries of lectures for easier group and individual study. If you do not like to study in groups, find another method that works for you. Maybe you need to go to a quiet place like the library or a coffee shop each night for a few hours. Maybe you need to make note-cards (by hand or digitally) for yourself. Find out what works for you and stick to it. Just remember that, above all, consistency is key.

One side note on how much students study: at this point in your academic career, you have self-selected yourself into a group of students that have done well in school. If one of your fellow students claims they never have to study, or that the material is a breeze, either completely ignore them, or understand that they are misrepresenting reality. Everyone studies, and everyone should. Do not feel bad that you are plugging away in the library while other students are "out on the town"—for every story you hear, there are countless other student hours spent studying as well.

Find a Way to Manage the Stress

When students struggle with the didactic portion of the PA program curriculum, this can impact nearly everything in their lives. Stress affects people in different ways, and you will need to find a way to balance the stress in your life as a PA student. For me, working out each day was a great way for me to deal with my stress, and I would even study while walking on the treadmill or the elliptical. Some PA students participate in sports teams together, while others plan social outings over the weekends.

Remember, your classmates are going through the same academic stresses that you are, so you may find that talking with a fellow student can be helpful for letting off some steam. Also, do not be afraid to reach out to family members or close friends if you need to vent about school. Having a plan in place to deal with the stress and a support system is important.

Whatever you do to cope the stress, remember to take care of yourself. Make sure you eat properly and try to get as much sleep as you can. If you are having trouble managing the course-load, speak to someone at your program about it. Your professors and advisers have dealt with overwhelmed students before, so they will likely be able to find you help if you need it. Many universities have counseling centers in place that PA faculty members can refer you to if necessary.

Sometimes the competition among PA students can be very intense. Most PA students are extremely intelligent, and they may be used to obtaining high marks in school. In nearly every PA program, there will be students who naturally excel when it comes to tests and grades. While it is important to do well in school, try hard to ignore the competition. You are in PA school to learn. So, try to do the best that you can without allowing your grades and the grades of your peers to upset you. Remember, when PA school is over and done, it will be you and your patient alone in the exam room, not you, your patient, and your classmates. Doing your personal best, as long as you pass, is all that will matter in the long run.

Get Organized

The best advice I can give you for surviving the didactic portion is to stay organized. Try to decide what is most important in terms of studying and manage your time wisely. You will never regret being well-prepared. You may also consider asking the faculty to help you stay organized—especially the course director or preclinical coordinator. These people have plenty of experience, and they are dedicated to helping you succeed in the program.

Follow the Rules

The most successful students are those that do what is asked of them and do not cause problems for other students or for faculty. There will be instances when you believe something is unfair (such as finding out you have an exam on material you just received a few hours before).

For the most part, unless you absolutely cannot live with something, I urge you to "suck it up" and deal with it. Remember, other students are suffering through the same stringent requirements that you are and they are not protesting. If you rock the boat with other classmates or faculty members (especially early on in the program), you may make your own life more miserable throughout the duration of your time in PA school.

I have known students who have alienated themselves among their peers, as well as students who have broken rules and delayed their own graduations. For example, some PA students will inevitably decide to "play hooky" during their clinical rotations, by missing days and/or lying to their preceptors about university training requirements.

These students often find themselves in serious trouble, as faculty members regularly communicate with preceptors about student attendance and performance. Keep this in mind: if there is a rule in place, it was created for a reason. Before you break a rule and make a costly mistake, politely discuss the issue with a faculty member. If you have a valid reason for potentially not abiding by a specific rule, it is best to address it with faculty as professionally as possible.

Use the Right (Correct) Resources

During the didactic portion, you will need the books that are required for your courses. Find out if any of the upperclassmen are willing to sell or share their books with you before you purchase them all on your own. It is also a good idea to ask your peers or colleagues which books they have found particularly useful before purchasing. Some books may be available for borrowing from the library or from the PA program itself.

To be successful in PA school (and, in life), you need to have the appropriate resources at hand. While in some instances you may be able to look information up online to get by, this is not the best method to get through PA school. Make sure you have the books you need for your courses available. Not having the necessary book can make studying much more difficult, and can ultimately hurt your grades and your success in the program. There are plenty of low-cost options for buying books. Be sure to review online sources and consider purchasing used books to reduce fees.

In addition to the required course reading, there are also a number of terrific books on medical and surgical topics that past students have relied on to assist with their learning. Below are some of the most helpful book series for studying and test-taking your didactic year. I urge you to go to a bookstore and thumb through them to see if purchasing one of them to assist you through a difficult topic may be worth the extra money.

- The Blueprints Series
- High-Yield Series
- First Aid Series
- Board Review Series
- Made Ridiculously Simple Series
- The Secrets Series

The Clinical Phase "Pearls"

Once you get to the clinical portion of the program, you have made it through the first gauntlet. Clinical rotations are in no way easy, but the stress of a clinical rotation is much more physical than it is mental—and most people appreciate that. Most schools have you participate in rotations that are approximately 4-8 weeks long. Each rotation will be a different specialty: for example, you may spend your first rotation doing family practice, and your next rotation doing general surgery. There are some rotations that you are required to do, and others that you may choose to participate in.

What you will actually be doing for each varies from rotation to rotation. Sometimes you will be working the dayshift, and other times you will be working night shifts. Try to adapt the best that you can. Most hospital rotations will include some type of morning rounds, followed by floorwork (drawing blood, ordering tests, etc.) or actually spending time in the operating room. If you are working in an outside clinic, you will likely be examining patients all day. Again, each rotation is unique in that it provides you with a different type of training, in a different setting, with different hours and responsibilities.

Some rotations will require you to travel great distances, which can make your day seem even longer. During my surgery rotation, I had to be at the hospital by 5 a.m. to "pre-round" on my patients. Because my rotation was so far away, I had to leave my house around 3:30 a.m. in order to be on-time. Unfortunately, this is not abnormal. You can expect to work long hours on your clinical rotations.

When I was a student doing a surgical rotation, I did not know what to expect. The first day of my first surgical rotation, I was told to scrub into a case in the operating room. Excitedly, I scrubbed in and gowned up just as I had learned in my PA class beforehand. What I was not prepared for, however, was the fact that the operation would last nearly six hours! About three hours into the case, I began to feel a little bit light-headed. I had never fainted before, so I thought I would be fine. A few minutes later, I felt even worse.

The next thing I remember was nurses giving me oxygen and tucking me into a recovery room bed. I had fainted in the operating room. While this is extremely embarrassing, it is not uncommon. PA students and medical students who are not used to being in the operating room for long periods of time are much more likely to get sick. However, you can prepare yourself. The secret is to keep a snack in your labcoat pocket and a beverage in your bag at all times. You never know when you will get a chance to eat on rotations, and having something handy can prevent you from getting sick or getting lightheaded.

If a hospital gives you anything to use while you are there, like a pager or a mobile device, I suggest you take very good care of it. You need not guard it with your life, but do treat it like your own. When I was a student, one of the hospitals required me to use their pager in addition to my own. One day, while I was going to the bathroom with my labcoat on the pager fell out of my pocket and into the toilet just as I flushed. My preceptors were very kind once they stopped laughing. Unfortunately, I did have to pay for a replacement pager because I had lost the original. So, be careful with other peoples' property. If you damage it or lose it, you will likely have to pay for it.

Rotation Terminology

There are some terms you should be familiar with before you begin your rotations. The first is "pimping." First guesses aside, pimping students on hospital rounds is actually the questioning practice physicians (and PAs) use to force students to be prepared and to think quickly. Attending physicians and physician assistants typically pimp students by asking them obscure questions while expecting students to respond with correct answers. When people pimp students, they *think* they are helping to teach them something; however, this method of making someone feel stupid because they do not remember exact details is not necessarily the best way to teach.

You may find that if you are put on the spot and asked to recite specific information that you do not know, you are more likely to remember it after looking it up later on. On the contrary, you may find that you have an unconscious desire to forget the information if the experience of being forced to regurgitate information was extremely traumatic.

Regardless of how this method impacts your learning, it is a common practice and you should be prepared for it.

Another term you should be familiar with is "scutwork," because as a PA student, you will definitely do your fair share of scutwork. Scutwork refers to a number of patient care activities that offer very little educational value for the student. For example, a PA student is doing scutwork if he is sent to deliver bloods to the lab, asked to transport a patient to another floor, or told to make phone calls for a resident or intern. Oftentimes they are tasks that need to be done in order to facilitate patient care, but tasks that offer very little in terms of learning experiences.

Hopefully, when you are a PA student, you will not be doing too much scutwork. However, if you find yourself in a position where you are getting plenty of scutwork but very little substantive experience, bring it to the attention of your preceptor or your program's administrators. Remember—you are paying to learn.

Adapting to Each New Environment can be Challenging

It may take a week or two before you fully understand what your role will be in the particular setting. I encourage you to create goals for the rotation early on and discuss these with your preceptor when you begin. This way, your preceptor has a general idea as to what you would like to learn during your time with them. While your preceptor may not be able to accommodate all of your educational goals, by keeping them informed, you are allowing them to assist you as much as they can.

In the hospital setting and in the outpatient setting you are likely to utilize different types of technology on a daily basis. As a student, this can be challenging—in some instances you are granted access to the electronic medical record programs; in others, you may be completely cut off from that access. Do your best to learn the basics about the different programs quickly so that you can be helpful to the clinicians you are working with. If you are not able to utilize the medical record system, do other tasks throughout the day to make yourself useful while your preceptors are charting. This may be a great time to get some practice with dictating (if opportunities exist), or with studying for your end of rotation examination.

Find a Way to Keep Yourself Comfortable

Spending long hours on your feet during rotations will require you to purchase a pair of good shoes. Regardless of your budget, it will not take long before you find yourself willing to submit to the expense of quality footwear. You may already have a personal preference when it comes to shoes, and if you do that is fine. Most people I know wear tennis shoes or special orthopaedic shoes. If you are looking to purchase a great (but expensive) pair of shoes, my colleagues recommend the following brands: Dansko, Skechers, Ecco, Birkenstock, and Merrell.

I recommend investing in at least one good pair of shoes for your rotations—if for nothing else in this book, you will someday thank me for this advice. You may also want to consider wearing compression stockings if you are standing for long periods. I have found that my legs and feet ache significantly less if I wear both compression stockings and comfortable shoes during the day.

Kill Them With Kindness

Try to make the best of your rotations; after all, this is the only clinical experience you are going to get before you are working on your own. Even if someone makes it clear that you are not wanted on a rotation (for example, another student or employee), do not take it personally. In fact, kill them with kindness. Demonstrate that you are the bigger person in the situation by performing your tasks with a smile.

(Do not misinterpret this: I am not encouraging you to be sarcastic or inappropriate by any means). Simply, work harder to show that you want to be there and that you want to learn as much as you can despite the other person's feelings about you being there. This way, they will have nothing bad to say about you in the end.

Be Assertive

If someone offers to teach you something, take them up on it. You should never refuse an opportunity to learn something new. As an example, a fellow PA student made an effort to keep in touch with the medical and surgical residents in some of the hospitals after he had finished his rotation. The residents informed him of any unique cases they had, and because of his curiosity and willingness to learn, he ended up seeing a lot of great medical and surgical cases. (Before doing this make sure it is approved by your PA program as some institutions have very specific guidelines regarding student credentialing).

Be On-Time

Being on-time actually means being early. Yes, this is a bit confusing. However, when it comes to clinical rotations, preceptors expect you to be there early—even if they do not tell you this. For example, if someone tells you to arrive at 7:00 AM, you should arrive at 6:45 AM. Plan accordingly and do not be lazy. If you have an accident or legitimate reason for being late, notify your preceptor immediately, and do not let it happen again. I have seen students fail rotations because of tardiness.

If you have a great attitude, and you are willing to get your hands wet (or dirty), you can learn an incredible amount on your clinical rotations. The best mantra I can give you about your rotations is: be on-time, work hard, smile, volunteer or read if you have downtime, and **do not whine!**

Finally, also write down contact information for physicians and other healthcare professionals whose company or work styles you enjoy. Even though I sound like a skipping CD, you may need letters of recommendation in the future, or you may want to network professionally. Keep your contact list current! PA school is tough, but once you complete your first rotation, you can complete them all—and you can certainly finish the program.

Part VI: Planning for a Career

Creating a Plan

After you have finished PA school, but before you begin looking for a job, you should take a moment—or an afternoon—to reconsider *why* you chose to practice medicine or surgery, and *what* you hope to get out of it. You may have chosen this profession because you want a satisfying and challenging career. You may have chosen this profession because you want to learn and gain experience and then move on to something else. Or, you could be in it for the money and the freedom that will provide for you and your family. Whatever your reasons are, having a clear understanding will make planning your career much easier, and will also help you develop measuring sticks to accurately chart your success along the way.

When it comes to career development, you, and only you, are ultimately responsible for what happens. If you work as a cardiothoracic physician assistant for two years and never learn to manage patients in the cardiac intensive care unit, then you are at least partly responsible for not having had that experience. The same holds true for a physician assistant who has spent two years working in family practice and still has trouble performing a pelvic exam. The skills you gain from these initial work experiences will help shape the PA that you will become and the type of practice you will enjoy or dislike.

At the beginning of your career, you have an opportunity to think about which direction you want your career to take. First, think about where you see yourself in a year or two—then, in five years. What do you hope to accomplish? Do you want to improve your procedure skills? Do you want to become specialized? Creating an idea about where you see your career heading will help you decide which direction you will take.

Thinking about these topics now will also save you from considering those same questions for the first time during a job interview. After you have thought through your answers, write them down and then

walk away. Come back after you have spent some time doing something completely different, and re-read your thoughts. Do they still
make sense? Would you be comfortable sharing them with someone
else you trusted? Would you be happy if this was the answer you
provided during a job interview? Refine your thoughts again, and then
take the opportunity to run them past a friend or colleague (or fellow
student). The ultimate result of your work will be a better, personal
understanding of what you want to do, and what others will understand
about what you want to do.

The first few years of clinical practice are important because, during
that time, you will develop work habits that will be much harder to
change later on. Your ability to perform a procedure or care for a
patient is often shaped by the "way it is done" in a particular office or
hospital. Your career will also be shaped by some of the people that
you work with during your first job. Think carefully about where you
want to learn new skills and from whom you want to learn these new
skills. Do not be embarrassed to ask your fellow colleagues about who
performs which procedure most successfully, and then ask that practitioner to demonstrate for you. Not only will you learn from the best,
you might make a friend or start developing a mentor relationship
simply by requesting help.

Deciding on a Work Setting

Selecting your first job can be difficult. As a new PA, and even after
some helpful career goal self-exploration, it can be hard to decide
which setting is best-suited for you. And while some people have no
problem figuring this out, PAs with varied interests in many areas can
find this decision to be overwhelming.

Nowadays, PAs work in almost every specialty imaginable, including
burn surgery, cardiothoracic surgery, colorectal, critical care, emergency medicine, family practice, general surgery, head and neck, ear nose
and throat, neurosurgery, ophthalmology, oncology, orthopedic surgery, pediatrics, plastic surgery, transplant surgery, urology, interven-
tional radiology, and so on. This is one of the greatest benefits of being
a PA: you do not have to specialize in one specific area! But it is also a

burden—too many choices can present as difficult a situation as too few.

So, how do you find a good fit for you? A good fit means that you have found a job for which you are well suited, in a setting that matches your long-term goals. A job that is well suited for you will allow you to utilize most of your skills, interests, and talents. By doing a little bit of prep work and having at least a basic understanding of what your goals are, you can find a job that is a good fit for you.

You will have to assess your interests, think about the different work settings, and then consider what each of these may be able to offer you. You also have to determine your long-term goals, and balance these with your immediate and long-term financial needs. The remainder of this chapter is filled with tools that will help you determine what type of physician assistant job might be best for you.

The following charts are meant to help you narrow your interests. The information listed is of course not all encompassing; it just provides a general overview and a way to focus your thoughts on some carefully-considered questions.

Assessment of Interest and Skill

I like or want to...	Yes	No	If yes, then consider working in...
Start work early in the morning			Hospital, Surgery or Private Practice
Start work later in the afternoon or evening			Hospital
Work a consistent schedule every day			Hospital or Private Practice
Work nights or weekends			Hospital or Per Diem
Work only a day or two per week			Hospital (Per Diem) or Private Practice (Per Diem)
To see patients on rounds with other physicians and PAs			Hospital or Internal Medicine Private Practice
To see patients on rounds by myself			Hospital, Internal Medicine (or other Specialty) or Private Practice
See fewer patients so I can take my time talking to patients			Hospital (Specialty), Private Practice (Specialty) or a Practice in a Rural Setting
See many patients throughout the day, each of them quickly			Hospital, Private Practice or Family Practice
Spend time documenting and billing			Private practice or Hospital (with Outpatient Clinic)
Stay in one office most of the day			Private practice
Stand or walk to different offices or floors most of the day			Hospital or Surgery
Dictate			Private Practice or Hospital
Perform complex procedures			Hospital (Surgery or Emergency Medicine)

Perform simple procedures			Family Practice, Private Practice (Family Practice or Specialty) or Hospital (Surgery or Emergency Medicine)
Learn general medicine			Family Practice or Hospital (Internal Medicine or Emergency Medicine
Be involved in managing rare conditions using cutting edge techniques			Major Teaching Hospital
Be involved in diagnosing rare conditions but transferring them to bigger hospitals			Rural Hospital
Have my own prescription pad			Private practice or Hospital (if working for one specific physician)
Make a lot of money			Specialty (Private Practice or Hospital) or Surgery (Night or Weekend Shifts)
Have good health benefits			Hospital (Also some Private Practice Settings – although not always consistent)
Have good retirement benefits			Hospital (Also some Private Practice Settings – although not always consistent)
Have a PA mentor to teach me			Hospital
Have a physician mentor to teach me			Private Practice
Interact with many people (non-patients) throughout the day			Hospital

Interact with only a core group of people (non-patients) each day			Private Practice (Clinic Only)
Perfect one specific procedure or area of medicine/surgery			Specialty
Become a chief or senior PA			Hospital
Transition my career into academia at some point			Hospital, Private Practice, Major Teaching Hospital
Work with several cutting-edge physicians			Major Teaching Hospital
Prescribe different drugs frequently			Hospital, Family Practice
Prescribe the same drugs frequently			Specialty Practice, Surgery
Create treatment plans mostly on my own			Family Practice, Private Practice or Specialty Practice (inpatient or outpatient)
Create treatment plans with the help of other PAs and physicians			Hospital, Specialty practice or Private Practice
Perform tasks delegated to me by other PAs or physicians			Hospital
Have a pager or mobile device provided			Hospital or Private Practice
Have my own office			Family Practice or Private Practice
Take some extra time to hone my skills with the guidance of other PAs and physicians			Residency or Fellowship

Once you have filled out this table, you will have a better idea of what type of setting you should consider. When you are seeking a job, you have to remind yourself to factor in your specific interests and needs because they can be easily lost in the excitement of interviews and applications. Of course, these tools are only here to help you narrow down your ideas and help determine which type of setting or job might be best for you.

Below, I have detailed a few of the main settings that PAs may work in: primary care, hospital, and specialty-private practice. I have identified some of the basic information about each of these settings so you can compare them and develop a personal understanding of which may be the best for you. As a full-time employee you will be spending a great deal of time in one particular setting. Think carefully about where you want to work before you even begin to apply for jobs.

Primary Care

Primary care settings are usually staffed by a supervising physician (or several), physician assistants, nurse practitioners, nurses, medical assistants, medical coding and billing specialists, transcriptionists, and front desk staff. Your primary responsibilities will be examining, diagnosing, and treating patients; writing referrals; writing prescriptions; documenting patient encounters; and billing.

Advantages
- Day shift
- Usually no weekends
- Busy – may see up to 50 patients a day
- One worksite
- May be easier to get vacation time, especially around holidays as office may be closed
- Autonomy in practice
- Wide range of medical conditions
- May offer loan repayment (if participates in the National Health Scholars Program)
- Will help solidify general medical knowledge

Disadvantages
- Billing
- Paperwork
- Limited to one worksite

- Vacation may be limited to when your supervising physician takes vacation
- If you are a salaried employee, you may work long hours without getting paid for your additional time
- Busy – 50+ patients per day can be a lot
- You may dislike your supervising physician
- You may not have the opportunity to participate in a 401(k) or 403(b) program
- You may work as an independent contractor and have to deal with your taxes personally

Hospital Setting

Hospital settings are usually staffed by physicians (both supervising and residents), nurse practitioners, physician assistants, nurses, and a variety of other healthcare employees. Your primary responsibilities will be participating in patient rounds; communicating with other team members; examining, diagnosing, and treating patients; ordering and interpreting laboratory and radiology tests, prescribing medications; documenting medical charts; and participating in procedures as necessary.

Advantages
- All types of work shifts available
- Often limited to one worksite
- Usually paid hourly, so you receive overtime pay if it is worked
- Often generous vacation time in contract
- Typically work with multiple physicians and physician assistants in a team
- Opportunities to work with students
- Typically offer generous healthcare and retirement plans
- Opportunities to switch positions within hospital system if other openings

Disadvantages
- Often required to work weekends and holidays
- You may be required to work on-call
- You may not have your own room or office

- Vacation may be limited by inadequate staffing to provide coverage
- Limited autonomy, as you are part of a clinical team

Specialty – Private Practice

Private practice specialty settings are usually staffed by a supervising physician (or several), nurse practitioners, physician assistants, nurses, medical assistants, medical coding and billing specialists, transcriptionists, and front desk staff. Your primary responsibilities will be examining, diagnosing, and treating patients; performing procedures; writing referrals; writing prescriptions; documenting patient encounters; and billing.

Advantages
- Day shift
- Often no weekend work (however, this depends on the practice setting)
- You likely will have your own room or office
- Opportunity to develop your own patients or clinics
- One worksite, although you may be required to travel to others
- May be easier to get vacation time, especially holidays as practice may be closed
- Opportunity to become skilled in a specific area of medicine or surgery
- Autonomy in practice

Disadvantages
- Billing and coding
- Paperwork
- If you are salaried, you may work long hours without extra pay
- Busy – you may see 50+ patients per day
- You may dislike your supervising physician
- Vacation may be limited to when your supervising physician takes vacation
- You may not have opportunity to participate in a 401(k) or 403(b) program
- You may not see a broad spectrum of medical issues

- Oftentimes very busy, especially if your supervising physician is in the operating room or clinic most days, leaving you as the only provider in the hospital or clinic

Sometimes, due to a lack of clear thinking or a need for money, physician assistants accept jobs that are a recipe for disaster. I made that mistake when I first began work as a new PA. I thought I wanted to work in private practice, so I first interviewed at a few different places, and then decided on a specialty private practice. After only a few short days, I realized I did not get along well with the physician I was working for. It did not take long for me to realize that I could not continue working in that environment and still maintain my sanity.

Within two weeks of working at my new job, I spoke to my supervising physician about how I felt. The physician apologized for making me feel uncomfortable, and offered me a raise if I would continue working there. I considered it. But, despite the offer of additional money, I concluded that I simply could not handle working in a place that I did not feel comfortable.

I learned from this experience that working in a setting with only one physician is difficult if the physician and you do not work well together. I decided that it would be best for me to work in a setting where there were multiple physicians to work with. I began looking for jobs in hospitals and was able to secure a position that was much more suited to my needs because I was able to work with multiple physicians and several other PAs.

My experience provided two lessons. First, it is difficult to make a good decision based on only a brief job interview. Second, if you are uncomfortable (and have the choice), leave. If you have opportunities to speak with other people who work in that particular practice, or hospital department, take those opportunities because they may be able to give you a better idea as to whether or not you will like working there. But also remember that, even though you have begun a job, if it is not a good fit for you, it is alright to consider leaving—and it is ok to leave! It is not worth your time to work somewhere that you will hate, especially when there are always great work opportunities for PAs out there.

Many physician assistant students garner job opportunities throughout their clinical rotations.   Remember to make every effort to treat a clinical rotation like a job interview, especially if you are interested in working in that site in the future. Accepting a job at a previous rotation site can be mutually beneficial for both you and the physician.   You have already had an opportunity to get to know the physician and staff you will be working with, and you know that you enjoyed your experience.   The physician benefits because he or she does not need to spend time searching for a PA and it may take a shorter period of time to train you.

Residencies and Fellowships: To Do or Not to Do?

While most physician assistant-school graduates go directly into practice after school, there are alternatives. Residencies and fellowships provide interested physician assistants with opportunities to obtain additional training in a specialized area of practice. This additional training is not required for most jobs, but there may be specific, highly-competitive positions (for example, a job in hand surgery) where residency or fellowship experience might give some clear advantages.

Postgraduate training programs are designed to be intense, and participants in a residency or fellowship gain a great deal of clinical skills and knowledge in a condensed period of time. Most postgraduate programs can be completed in 12-15 months, although some programs are longer in length and may go even deeper into the subject material of the program's focus.

These types of programs often provide the participant with a salary or stipend, healthcare benefits, vacation time, and even time off for continuing medical education conferences. Additionally, nearly every program provides a certificate of completion, and some programs also include a Masters degree when the program is successfully completed. (Those programs that include a Masters degree also require tuition fees for the degree).

The following are the "pros" for considering postgraduate training:

- Developing more confidence in clinical skills – essentially, paid clinical training
- Opportunities to see complex clinical cases
- Opportunities to work with and network with other PAs and MDs in the specialty of your choosing
- Following completion of residency, you will likely start at higher salary than a new graduate
- When transitioning, this may be an opportunity for an experienced PA to change specialty areas if her clinical practice has been limited to one area

While the benefits are many, the accreditation process is only now catching up with physician assistant residency and fellowship programs. Since accreditation is optional, the option was just proposed in 2007, and the process to become accredited is costly and lengthy, it is unlikely that every program will be accredited—at least for several years. However, accreditation is just one small part of a program's value, and should not be the determining factor in your analysis, as that consideration is currently not a focus of the profession.

Physician assistant residencies are available in the following specialties: cardiothoracic surgery, critical care, dermatology, emergency medicine, hospitalist medicine, neonatology, neurology, neurosurgery, OB-GYN, oncology, orthopedics surgery, psychiatry, rheumatology, sleep medicine, surgery, trauma, and urology. There are also teaching fellowships available for physician assistants that want to gain experience for a career in academia.

For a current list of the current PA residencies and fellowships, please review the Association of Postgraduate Physician Assistant Programs' ("APPAP") website: http://www.appap.org. You should also review the Index of Residencies and Fellowships located at the end of this book.

After reviewing the APPAP website for the current list of residencies and fellowships, contact the programs directly for even more information. And while several of the programs have websites to review, the absolute most current and informed information you will get will come from direct inquiries to the program directors. An e-mail to a provided contact could let you know about un-posted or unpublicized opportunities, or whether there are particulars that can help your application. I advise you to ask lots of questions and try to make a very informed decision about whether or not a specific residency program is right for you.

The application process can be daunting (although not as bad as CASPA!), so review all of the appropriate information before you begin to apply. Additionally, if you are a competitive applicant, you should prepare to travel to the site for an interview (this may require you to take time off from school or work).

Considerations for residency selection:

- Look for a balance between didactic and clinical training – consider how much time you will be spending in the classroom versus how much time you will be spending participating in the clinical setting. A good residency will have a workable mix of both, enabling you to learn as much as possible.
- Work hours – many residency programs limit the number of hours a PA is allowed to work each week. Does your program abide by these limitations (or at least say it does)?
- Location – can you imagine living in the location for a year or more?
- Stipend / Salary – does the residency or fellowship provide you with enough to live on? You may be able to defer your student loans during the program, if you have them.
- Vacation – does the program allow time off? You will be working very hard; is the provided vacation time going to be enough for you? For reference, most programs range from 2-4 weeks of vacation time per year.
- Subsidized housing/family housing – are there opportunities to live in subsidized housing? If you have a significant other, or children, are there any discounted options for family housing?

If you decide to participate in a residency or fellowship, I am confident you will find it a valuable experience. As more and more PAs are working in specialties, obtaining advanced postgraduate training will make you more competitive by enhancing your ability to find a job and practice in the specialty of your choice—and the opportunity you will have immediately after you graduate, before setting down too many "roots," is ideal for this type of experience.

Flexible Work Arrangements

One of the most appealing aspects about the physician assistant profession is the fact that not every physician assistant works a 9-5 job. There are flexible work arrangements available for those people who want to balance the competing demands of a career and other priorities. PAs may want a reduced-hour work schedule so they can spend more time with their families or for other personal reasons. A high demand for healthcare professionals has encouraged employers to be more receptive to flexible work schedules. The healthcare profession cannot afford to lose experienced physician assistants, especially when the costs of finding, hiring, and training new employees are extremely high.

Flexible work arrangements can include any type of part-time, per Diem, or contract work (locum tenens) schedules. There are many types of flexible opportunities available for physician assistants all over the United States, and even some abroad. The hourly pay rate may be higher than it would be with a traditional work schedule; however, higher hourly pay may be offset by decreases in healthcare and retirement benefits.

Timing is also a large part of determining your work schedule. If you are a brand-new employee and decide to reduce your work schedule, your employer may not be very receptive. An inexperienced physician assistant should spend the first few years out of school trying to learn how to be a PA, not trying to minimize work demands.

If you have been working for an employer for a few years and wish to reduce your work hours to part-time, *then* you should bring up the topic. Many physicians and institutions are willing to work with you if you have developed a good working relationship. Here, planning and presentation will be key. Instead of an offhand request for a different schedule, carefully consider exactly what you wish to do and how this will impact your workplace. Develop a clear, professional plan for your hours, and schedule a meeting to present that plan to your supervisor.

Use that opportunity to demonstrate how your current work will be unaffected, or (even better) how this will improve service. And remember, an institution or a private practice also benefits by having a satisfied physician assistant working for it. These benefits include better health, and a loyal employee who is grateful for the opportunity to re-arrange his or her schedule.

Contract Work

Contract jobs for physician assistants have gained fairly wide acceptance. Some hospitals and private practice physicians use contract physician assistants to fill employment needs while they look for someone full-time, or simply to a cover maternity or medical leave. Contract work is a great option for physician assistants who want to work for a period of time and then pursue other interests.

Contract work may allow physician assistants who are parents to spend more time at home with their children, while still working intermittently. Contract work may also be an option for a new physician assistant who has been unsuccessful in finding a full-time job. Physician assistants who want to travel may decide to take a contract job in another part of the country for a few months. The reasons for choosing to do contract work are endless, just like available opportunities.

Although contract work does work best for some people, it may not include healthcare or retirement benefits. If opt for contract work, be sure that you and the hospital (or outside company) are clear about what your responsibilities will be, what your pay rate will be, and how long the contract will be in effect for.

Per Diem Work

Per Diem work is another option for physician assistants who are looking to work, but desire (or require) a more flexible schedule.

Hospitals and private practices use per Diem physician assistants to work shifts that they are unable to cover, to fill in employment needs as they arise, or to work nights or weekends when the full-time staff members are not "on the clock." Per Diem work is a great option for physician assistants who are parents and want to spend more time at home with their families. Per Diem work is also a great option for those people who work a full-time job, but are looking to pick up additional shifts. Many PAs working in academia also work in per Diem clinical jobs to help maintain their clinical skills. Typically, employers require per Diem employees to work one or two shifts a month—which can easily be done in addition to a full time job.

Per Diem employees are usually paid a reasonable, hourly rate because these jobs do not typically include healthcare or retirement benefits. Per Diem jobs may also include a weekend or night shift pay differential. If you consider per Diem work, consider all your options, and balance the type of work offered with the schedule, pay, and your "feel" for the workplace.

The Most Important Steps: Passing the PANCE and Getting a License

In order to practice as a PA, you must be a credentialed PA-C ("Physician Assistant Certified"), or, in the state of New York, a RPA-C (Registered Physician Assistant Certified). To become credentialed, you must successfully pass the Physician Assistant National Certifying Exam ("PANCE"), a computerized, multiple-choice test that every PA must take. The exam is comprised of 360 questions that cover topics in both medicine and surgery. It is a very challenging exam that will require you to study a great deal beforehand.

First, you must register for the PANCE. You may do so online before you graduate, through the National Commission on Certification of Physician Assistants ("NCCPA") website. Their website address is: http://www.nccpa.net.

If you register before you graduate, you must provide the NCCPA with release information so that your school can send the NCCPA appropriate information explaining that (a) you are in good standing and (b) you will graduate from the program—this is called a letter of eligibility. Once this process is complete, you will be assigned a "window" test opportunity. This testing window allows you to register to take the exam anytime within a specific period of time, and you will select a testing center and a date of examination. Be careful when selecting a date and location—if you need to make a change to either, it can be both complicated and costly. (Currently, the NCCPA allows you to make changes up to 24 hours before the day of the scheduled exam). Most students need close to a month of full-time study to prepare; but those students who are exceptional test-takers (or think they are) may decide they only need two or three weeks before taking the examination. Make the decision based on your specific educational, financial, and work circumstances.

Once you have arranged a time and location, start studying for the PANCE. Be realistic in your study goals, keeping in mind that this exam is extremely difficult, and it is not uncommon for one or two students out of every graduating class to fail. While your goal is to pass the exam, if you do fail it is not the end of the world—you are allowed to retake the test. But to do so, you will have to repay the application fee, and then wait to register for another testing window (which means you will wait at least 90-or-so days before testing again).

In order to help students study for the PANCE, the NCCPA has designed "blueprints" to guide you. These blueprints can be found on the NCCPA website, and these blueprints describe the different areas of content on the exam. For example, approximately 16% of the exam questions will deal with patient history taking and performing physical examinations. The current blueprints available from the NCCPA website are listed below. Review the listed blueprints, but also (and always) check the information available online when you prepare, as the content is periodically updated. Then, print the current blueprints out to use as a guide for your studying.

Current Blueprints divided by Organ System:
    Cardiovascular: 16%
    Pulmonary: 12%
    Endocrine: 6%
    EENT (Eyes, Ears, Nose, Throat): 9%

Gastrointestinal / Nutritional 10%
Genitourinary: 6%
Musculoskeletal: 10%
Reproductive: 8%
Neurologic System: 6%
Psychiatry / Behavioral: 6%
Dermatologic: 5%
Hematologic: 3%
Infectious Diseases: 3%_____
Total of 100%

Current Blueprints divided by Task Areas:
History Taking and Performing Physical Examinations: 16%
Using Laboratory and Diagnostic Studies: 14%
Formulating Most Likely Diagnosis: 18%
Health Maintenance: 10%
Clinical Intervention: 14%
Pharmaceutical Therapeutics: 18%
Applying Basic Science Concepts: 10%_____
Total of 100%

The NCCPA website also offers an online Self-Assessment practice examination. The practice exam is an abbreviated version of the PANCE (it contains about half the questions), but completing the practice exam is an excellent way to prepare for the actual test. However, the feedback you will receive from the NCCPA is somewhat vague: you will not get to review the answers to each question, but you will receive an overview of your strengths and weaknesses. Once you register with the NCCPA, you will also gain access to the Self-Assessment program, which will. This program costs $35 per exam. Use these resources. The more you practice, and the more exposure to questions and test-like renditions you have, the better prepared you will be when you take the actual exam.

In PA school, you will likely take (or have taken) a "practice PANCE" called the ePackrat. The ePackrat is similar to the PANCE insofar as it is computerized and given in multiple-choice format. If your PA Program allows you to print and review the questions from the ePackrat, do it, and review your questions and answers. Using the ePackrat to help your PANCE preparation by printing out the sample questions from your ePackrat is a shortcut every PA should use because, as with the online PANCE practice exams, this will help develop your comfort level with the PANCE.

There also are several great study guides out there for the PANCE exam, although some of those programs come with a steep cost. You may want to consider sharing books or programs with classmates to save money, borrowing books from PAs who have already taken the exam, or hunting for used materials online. (You may even find useful review books to check out in your university's or hospital's library)

When studying for your exams in PA school, you were probably able to determine which method of studying worked best for you. (For me, working through practice questions was the most practical way for me to learn the material) But, I know other students who found attending a PA review course or reviewing each body system thoroughly worked best.

I think the best approach to studying, involves using multiple methods and sources—and, for the PANCE, this is an opportunity to return to your strengths when it comes to your primary study method; but to try something new as well. While your success will ultimately rely on how you learn best, you will be surprised at what you pick up if you try a new method of study—and you might be additionally motivated if you are trying something outside of your comfort zone.

PANCE Study Guides

Below, I have outlined some of the most common study guides, along with a description of each. Before purchasing anything, read product descriptions and reviews online—most of these items are frequently updated to keep content current. And, of course, there are additional guides available that I have not listed here.

Online PANCE study guides

- Med-Challenger (http://www.chall.com)
    - The Med-Challenger program is completely online, with over 4,700 practice questions with detailed answers, including over 3,400 images to review.
    - The program also provides Category I CME (although you cannot use these unless you are already a certified PA).
    - The approximate cost is $595.
- Kaplan Q bank online (http://www.kaplanmedical.com)
    - The Kaplan Q bank is an online program with over 1,200 practice questions with detailed answers.
    - The format is similar to the NCCPA.
    - The approximate cost is $100-$200 depending on the duration of access you purchase.
- McGraw Hill's PA Easy (http://www.paeasy.com)
    - PA Easy is an online program with 1,200 practice questions with full explanations.
    - The questions were written by PA faculty members.
    - The approximate cost is $79-$139 depending on the duration of access you purchase.
- Datachem software for PAs (http://www.datachemsoftware.com/pacprep.htm).
    - The Datachem software is a CD-based program with approximately 840 questions and detailed answers.
    - The approximate cost is $170.

Books used for the PANCE

- *A Comprehensive Review for the Certification and Recertification Examinations for Physician Assistants: Published in collaboration with AAPA and PAEA,* by Claire Babcock O' Connell and Sarah F. Zarbock
    - This study guide includes a 300 question pre-test and a 300 question post-test (available via a companion website).

- The book provides content review on each of the topics identified on the NCCPA Blueprints.
- The approximate cost is about $50. (In my opinion, the book is well worth the money).
- *Lange Q&A Physician Assistant Examination,* by Anthony A. Miller, Albert F. Simon, and Rachel Carlson
  - This book is a study guide with approximately 1300 practice questions and a CD-ROM for use in an electronic format for "test-like" conditions.
  - The approximate cost is $50.
- *Physician Assistant Board Review: Certification and Recertification with online exam simulation,* by James Van Rhee
  - This book is provides a companion website making it an interactive study guide with three different 300-question tests (a total of 900 questions) to take.
  - The approximate cost is $50.
- *Physician Assistant Exam Review: Pearls of Wisdom*, by Daniel Thibodeau and Scott Plantz
  - This book is meant to be used in a slightly different way than traditional review books.
  - The questions are short and to the point, with the answers right underneath the questions (no flipping to the back).
  - The book has over 4,300 "rapid-fire" questions for you to review.
  - The approximate cost is $40.
- *Davis's PA Exam Review: Comprehensive Guide to PANCE and PANRE Exams*, by Morton Diamond
  - The book is set-up with an "essentials" section where you can review key topics, and a "performance" section where you can take practice questions on those topics.
  - The book comes with a companion CD with additional practice questions. (But beware, book reviewers have noted that the companion CD does not work properly on Mac computers)
  - The approximate cost is $35.

Review Courses

- CME Resources (http://www.cmeresources.com)
    - This seminar is offered several times a year in different areas of the country.
    - The program offers review lectures on important topics for the PANCE, as well as hundreds of practice test questions for you to review.
    - Courses are generally 5 days long.
    - The approximate cost is $840.
- Certified Medical Educators (http://www.certifiedmedicaleducators.com)
    - This program is a 3-day comprehensive PANCE/PANRE review that is offered several times a year in different areas of the country.
    - The program covers the content on the NCCPA Blueprints, and also offers workshops if you wish to participate in hands-on activities.
    - The approximate cost is $425.
- UMDNJ Physician Assistant Certification & Recertification Examination Review Course (http://www.mycme.com/eproduct/5825)
    - This program can be downloaded online for a fraction of the cost of actually attending. And, the online program can be purchased as a whole or by individual body system.
    - The content includes lectures to watch and practice tests to take following the lectures.
    - The online program costs approximately $275. (There is, of course, a live course each year, if you are more motivated by sitting in lectures in-person—but the cost is substantially higher)
- Emory University Home Study Board Review DVD Course (http://emorypa.org/pa_board_review.htm)
    - This DVD program includes lectures that can be downloaded to your smartphone for easy access.
    - The DVD contains lectures, PDF handouts, and practice tests. Additionally, the program includes a 2-week

subscription to ExamMaster Online (allowing the
student to take even more practice questions). Emory
University also offers a live four-day conference once a
year as well.

- The DVD home study program costs approximately
$360.

Not all study guides are equal. When I took the PANCE, I found that I
did quite well on some practice tests and quite poorly on others. This is
not uncommon, as some programs are more difficult than others.
Again, your best course is to use a variety of study tools—in a variety
of formats—to become familiar with different formats and types of
questions. The following checklist will help you organize the material
I have presented thus far. Write down your progress, and try to organize your schedule.

PANCE Study Checklist

To-Do Before Taking the PANCE	Planned (date)	Completed (date)
Pay Fee (example)	*March, 2013*	*March 31, 2013*
Pay Fee		
Select Date and Location		
Print Blueprints from NCCPA Website		
Print out Copy of your ePackrat Test (if you can)		
Take NCCPA Practice Exam to Identify Weak Areas		
Purchase Study-Guide Book(s) or Program(s)		
Practice Questions – Score Greater than >70% on most tests		
Arrange for Good Night's Sleep and Breakfast before the Exam		

Be prepared for a long day at the testing center. The PANCE takes
approximately six hours (although, if you are a very quick test taker, it
is possible that you could end sooner than that). The testing center has
many rules—and while some of them are silly (like no gum-chewing),
all of them were in place for ostensibly good reasons.

You must bring two forms of photo identification with you, you must have your photo taken on-site, and you must have your palm scanned before you are even allowed to enter the exam room. You will have a locker that you can put your valuables in, and you may also keep beverages or snacks in the locker. (I would encourage you to take advantage of this option, as you will probably need to re-fuel or re-hydrate at least once during the exam).

Within the past five years, the NCCPA has changed the testing center company that it works with. The previous testing company caused many students problems, myself included. My experience was quite miserable and ended with me close to tears mid-exam. During one of the scheduled test breaks I went to my locker to get a piece of gum. While doing so, I was notified by a proctor from the testing center that I was not allowed to go to my locker, but only to the bathroom, and that because I had broken the rules my test would be invalid. I was not the happiest test-taker at that point. The woman then took a moment to review the rules and determined that, in fact, I *was* allowed to go to my locker. Lesson learned: practice enough that your understanding of the material is *so* solid that the unknowns of the test day will not derail all of your hard work.

Thankfully, I had studied enough before the exam, and had taken enough practice tests that my test-taking mechanics were automatic. I was able to complete the questions, and I finished my exam, but after my interaction with the proctor, I was certainly much more nervous and frustrated than I was before I began.

This raises a serious point: to avoid any problems at your testing facility, follow the rules. Make sure you read the exam tutorial that is provided at the testing facility before you begin your exam—and, in an abundance of caution, ask permission to do anything before you do it. While my test situation turned out fine, learn from my experience—you do not want to end up like me, and more stress to your test than necessary!

As with any exam, be sure to get a good night's sleep and to eat a good breakfast beforehand. Do not try new foods the day or morning before, and consider taking your final 8-12 hours before the exam off.

While last-minute cramming may be part of your study plan, it is not necessarily helpful. Many students close their last study book around dinner-time the night before the exam, and do their best to get their mind off the exam. (I suggest watching a movie or a television show (think comedy) and do your best to take the opportunity to relax).

Licensing

Each U.S. State requires that health professionals (with various titles) hold a license to practice. The act of licensing health professionals began in the 1800's, and each state has the authority and responsibility to restrict medical practice to those who are licensed.[40] The licensure process could be easy—or could be quite tedious, depending on which state you live in. The process can be quite timely as well. You may be lucky enough to get your license within a few weeks, or you may be unlucky and get held up somewhere along the way, in which the process can take months. (I have been "lucky" enough to have experiences with both, and neither is uncommon).

Most states will allow you apply for a license before you have actually passed the PANCE. To begin, you must fill out all of the application information, and send it to your appropriate state along with the necessary fee. But beware: some of the applications can be very lengthy. If you are unsure which state you will be practicing in, you may apply for more than one license—but of course this will add additional cost and time.

When completing one state license application, take one additional step that I guarantee will pay off future dividends: make a separate file (on paper or electronically) and keep list all the information you collect for the application. This "core" personal file will be invaluable the next time you apply for a different application, and might also help if you have to complete any other short or long-form applications. Think "Super Resume," one that includes more explicit information than you would normally provide: such as the precise dates you apply or are

---

[40] Davis, A. Your Physician Assistant State License. *PA Professional.* April 2011, page 6. Available at: http://paprofessional.cadmus.com/Index.aspx. Accessed on August 22, 2011.

accepted to programs, or when you take (and pass) the PANCE. You should also make a copy of your application before you submit it; some states will bounce your application back several times if there are any issues, and you want to be prepared to address every state question with the right information in front of you.

Many states also require fingerprinting and criminal background checks. Be sure to follow the guidelines as precisely as possible. If you live in the state you are applying to for licensure, you may be able to obtain a "Live Scan" fingerprint (inkless, electronic fingerprinting). However, if you are out-of-state, you may need to go to the local Sheriff's office and get fingerprinted the old-fashioned way. Regarding the clinical background check, you should find out which agency the state would like you to use to obtain this before attempting to get it on your own. Sometimes there are very specific instructions—inform yourself of these before you waste any time or money.

Your PA program must send in documentation indicating that you have met the successful requirements for completing the program. So, remember to notify your PA program of which states you are applying for licensure in, so that they can submit your appropriate information in a timely manner.

Once you have passed the PANCE, you must submit a request for NCCPA to send a copy of your scores to your state's licensing board. You can find out the specific information that your state requires by logging onto your state's website.

You may also need to provide verification of other held licenses. For example, if you had a professional license before becoming a physician assistant (for example, nursing or dental hygienist), you will probably need to contact that licensing agency and have the agency provide verification that you are (or were) in good standing. Again, once you collect this information, document what you learn in your separate "Super Resume" file.

It is possible to apply for more than one state license at a time. If you are unsure which state you will be living in or practicing in, you are allowed to apply for multiple licenses. (For example, I currently have two different state licenses). However, each license application will take time and money in order to process.

Additionally, many states require a "delegation to practice" form that must be completed by a supervising physician. You can oftentimes obtain a license to practice before you have the delegation agreement completed (so you can apply for a license even if you do not have a job yet). However, before you begin practicing as a PA in your new state, you should determine whether or not you need to have this agreement sent in to the state licensing agency. If you work at a hospital, they will likely facilitate this. However, if you work in a private setting, you will need to discuss this with your supervising physician before you begin working.

Never, Ever Lie on your License Applications

I have a friend who had (unfortunately) received a DUI (driving under the influence) ticket before beginning PA school. All of the licensing applications specifically ask if you have had any prior run-ins with the law. My friend was contemplating not mentioning the DUI on the application as she was concerned that it might hinder her ability to obtain her PA license. However, she consulted with a lawyer who informed her that it would be exceedingly unwise to omit something like that, especially considering most states perform criminal back-ground checks. While not numerous, there are stories of PAs who took a shortcut on their applications and, years later, when the omission or inaccuracy was discovered, the PAs were vulnerable to termination. Do not let that be you.

And, when planning your career, remember that obtaining any type of licensure takes time. You should allow an average 4-6 weeks for processing your new state license as some states may take longer and others may take a shorter period of time. The important thing is that you apply as early as possible so that you can obtain your license to practice as soon as you can.

Obtaining a DEA License

The Drug Enforcement Agency ("DEA") provides an opportunity for PA-Cs to obtain a special license to prescribe narcotic medications. While the DEA license is optional, you should consider getting it. It took a long time for our profession to obtain the opportunity to even apply for DEA licensing, and now that you have the opportunity, take advantage. But, the DEA license is a privilege—and an expensive one at that. Be forewarned that the cost of a new DEA license will run more than $550 for three years. And, despite what I said above, regardless of the benefits, the DEA license is not necessary in all practice environments and may not be worth the cost for you.

You can find out more information about obtaining a DEA license at the following website: http://www.deadiversion.usdoj.gov/

Changing Your Name or Address

After I got married, I had to change my name. While I was initially apprehensive, in the end it was much easier than I thought it was going to be. To get started, simply look up the necessary agencies online and send in the appropriate documentation. It can take 2-4 weeks for the paperwork to be processed. If you do have to change your name or address, please allow the agencies enough time to update your information before starting a new job.

Here are a few of the organizations you may need to contact if you have to make a personal information change:

- NCCPA (http://www.nccpa.net/)
- DEA (http://www.deadiversion.usdoj.gov/)
- AAPA (http://www.aapa.org/)
- Your state licensing board
- Your state PA organization
- Any other PA organizations you are a member of

Finding and Securing a Job

Once you determine which type of job setting might work best for you, it is time to start looking for a job. You may find a job through a posting online, through a previous rotation, through a PA journal, or even through word of mouth. When I first started looking for jobs, I used the internet to search certain websites every day. There are plenty of online sources to peruse; however, here are those websites I found most useful:

PA Job Link – Health-e-Careers
http://www.aapa.org
This website is sponsored in part by the AAPA, and you can find a link to this page at the AAPA website (in the "Find a Job" section). This is also a great website for national jobs, and it is frequently updated.

PA World
http://www.paworld.net
This is a comprehensive job website for physician assistants; however, it is not the most user-friendly. This website is updated daily, so I recommend checking it frequently. While you should absolutely use the site, I have found that old postings tend to linger on this site, so you may see a job listing that has already been filled.

PA Exchange
http://www.pa-exchange.com
This website displays jobs for both physician assistants and nurse practitioners. The website is updated frequently, and can be filtered by location—making it very helpful whether you have one location in mind, or are considering several.

United States Federal Government Jobs
http://www.usajobs.gov
This website is a great resource to look for physician assistant jobs all over the country. Some jobs are through the Veterans Affairs Department, while others are through the Health and Human Services Department. There are a variety of jobs posted, and they are updated frequently.

National Health Service Corp
http://nhsc.hrsa.gov

If you are specifically looking for a job that might offer loan repayment, you may want to check out the National Health Service Corp ("NHSC") website. There are many jobs for physician assistants interested in primary care on this website. The jobs are most often located in rural areas or urban underserved communities. As I write this, a two-year service commitment at a NHSC worksite will provide $60,000 towards loan repayment.

If you have a specific job interest—for example, you are looking for a PA job in cardiothoracic surgery—you should probably seek help from a specialty organization, such as the Association of Physician Assistants in Cardiovascular Surgery ("APACVS") or the American Association of Surgical Physician Assistants ("AASPA"). Both of these organizations post jobs frequently on their websites, as do many other specialty organizations. (You can find a comprehensive list of these organizations and their websites in the Index section of the book)

For local job postings, head to your state-sponsored PA organization's website (you can find a comprehensive list of these organizations and their websites in the Index section of the book). I have found these websites to be extremely useful in finding local jobs. Oftentimes you must be a member of the organization in order to view the job postings, but if you are going to be living in that area you should consider joining, both to network and to learn more about issues that concern PAs working in that particular state.

Some states even have specific chapters that divide the different state regions, and you may be able to join one of those groups as well. When I was moving out-of-state, I joined the state PA organization and discovered there was a specific group of physician assistants dedicated to the county I was moving to. I immediately contacted the group's leader and was added to their e-mail listserv. I found it to be extremely helpful, as the group regularly sent out job postings and information about local conferences.

Do not forget to check for job postings at your PA program, as former students often inform PA programs of job openings. If you are looking for a job in a different state than your current PA school, consider contacting PA schools near where you hope to work. They might just put you in touch with the right person.

You should also check hospital websites. Just as with fellowships, if you know you want to work at a certain hospital, you should contact the human resources department of the hospital directly to inquire about opportunities. Many times the hospital has openings that it has not posted on its website or advertised in any way yet. In some instances, the human resources contact will allow you to e-mail or fax a resume to them directly. And, of course, it never hurts to make a personal visit, as there is something special about meeting with a person face-to-face. You may want to consider hand-delivering a resume to the hospital you are interested in working at and asking them to keep it on file for future opportunities.

Do not overlook the value of going to continuing medical education ("CME") meetings and networking! At a CME conference, there are plenty of opportunities to meet new PAs and to make possible employment connections. In fact, there are often local hospitals and recruiters on-site who may try to entice you without much effort on your part.

Some physician assistants decide to work directly with a job recruiter. (For more information on this, search the internet for "physician assistant job recruiter"). A job recruiter will probably ask you to submit a resume, and then she will present you with a few job opportunities that may be of interest to you. Recruiters often work for agencies that are hired directly by healthcare institutions or physicians.

The advantage of using a recruiter is that they may make the job search and application process a breeze—they may even help you fill out the state license forms and credentialing paperwork. They are hired by their employers fill jobs fast, so they want to speed things up while trying to identify the best candidate for the job. A recruiter can be helpful if you are looking for a job in a location that is unfamiliar to you. But keep in mind that a recruiter's primary responsibility is to the employer, and not to you, and while your interests and talents are a part of the selection calculus, the recruiter wants to fill the job—not just make you happy. And, recruiters are required to weed through a lot of applicants, and you may be one of the applicants that did not make the cut.

Also, beware—in some instances the recruiter was hired because the institution or physician was unable to find a physician assistant to fill the position on their own. This means there might be something undesirable about the job—so make sure that you have reviewed all of the job's details before signing on the dotted line.

Do not forget about traditional job posting places. You may see something that sparks your interest in the back of a PA journal or newsletter, and many hospitals and private practices are "old school" and advertise solely in magazines and journals. Perusing classified ads in the local newspaper may also offer a few leads. And, although it may not be completely traditional, I would also review Craigslist (http://craigslist.org). I have obtained legitimate job interviews through Craigslist, but I would encourage you to proceed with caution when applying to jobs through this site as not all of the information provided is always accurate.

I think the most important thing to remember about searching for a job is that you need to let people know you are looking. You may have a friend or colleague who has learned of a PA position that may be of interest to you. Although it may seem awkward, do not be afraid to advertise your interests and skills to those around you. Word-of-mouth advertising works!

Many people I know have obtained interviews for jobs through friends. For example, one of the resident physicians I worked with during a clinical rotation contacted me several months later, letting me know about a great physician she worked with who was in need of a PA. In a similar fashion, I have connected many students pursing PA jobs with my own friends and colleagues who may have informed me of specific opportunities. You may be surprised by the number of people willing to help you land your first job—but first, you have to ask for help and market your skills a little bit.

Of course, there are exceptions, and people may randomly seek you out! Recently, I was at the gym and was wearing a t-shirt that said "Physician Assistant" on it. A woman approached me and inquired about my shirt. She then proceeded to ask me if I was looking for a job as she was a family practice physician and was hoping to hire a PA. Unfortunately, I was not looking for a job at the time; however, I did take her contact information in case I (or anyone I knew) was looking for a job in the future.

Creating a Cover Letter

When applying for a job, you should always send a cover letter. A cover letter gives you the opportunity to introduce yourself and explain your interest in the position you are applying for in your own words, without the added pressure of an in-person interview. Be sure the letter is brief and provides some insight about you that cannot easily be gathered from a quick look at your resume. For example, you may want to describe why you might be relocating to a particular city, or why you think you are good fit for a particular specialty. In the cover letter you should always include your current contact information, and be sure to address the hiring physician or recruiter by name, if known. I have included a copy of a sample cover letter to help guide you in creating your own:

Jane Doe, PA-C

Your address
Your phone number
Your e-mail

Date

Re: Application for Employment

Dr. Smith:

My name is Jane Doe, and I am a recent graduate of (your school's) physician assistant program. I would like to speak with you regarding the possibility of working as a physician assistant in your primary care practice.

As you will see from my enclosed resume, I have experience in a variety of clinical settings. I have completed ten months of clinical rotations during my training, four of which were focused on primary care. During these clinical rotations, I examined adult and pediatric patients in clinic and hospital settings, diagnosed conditions, wrote progress notes, and created treatment plans. I am comfortable performing different office procedures, including EKGs, phlebotomy, IV catheter insertion, injections, and skin biopsies.

I would enjoy speaking with you further regarding this job opportunity. Please contact me by telephone or e-mail to set up a personal interview.

Sincerely,

Your name

Anytime you send any material for a job, always make sure you have checked the spelling and punctuation. And, while it seems silly (you are a PA, not a proofreader), sending a cover letter or resume with obvious errors can absolutely cost you a job opportunity. An employer might decide that, if you have difficulty spelling the words on your cover letter correctly, how can she be sure you will not make spelling mistakes when you are writing patient prescriptions? Make sure you use the spell-check function on the computer to review your documents, in addition to printing them out and having someone else review them. Do not forget to do this—it is extremely important!

Creating a CV or Resume

First, make sure you know the difference between a curriculum vitae ("CV") and a resume. A CV acts as a complete record of your professional history, while a resume is a shorter, focused list of skills and work experience that quickly demonstrates how you can benefit a workplace.

In the United States, most people use the two interchangeably. However, you should always pay attention to whether the specific job you are applying to requires a CV or a resume, and try to tailor your document to their requests. In fact, if you are performing a broad job search, you should create one of each.

Creating a resume is one of your most important tasks when job hunting. A resume is the first opportunity that a physician or hospital has to decide whether or not they want to invite you for an interview. Research suggests that employers spend less than 30 seconds reviewing a resume, so yours needs to be organized and concise.[41] You do not want to be denied an interview simply because your resume was poorly done.

Great resumes are clear and simple. As a new grad, you should attempt to limit your CV or resume to one page. After you have experience as a PA (or if you have an extensive work history before becoming a PA), your CV or resume may exceed one page. Your first PA resume should include the following information:

- Name
- Contact information (make sure it is current)
- Education

---

[41] Dahring, R. Your Journey is Just Beginning. *Advance for NPs & PAs*. April 2011. Volume 2: Issue 4: Page 39-42. Available at: www.advanceweb.com/NPPA. Accessed August 22, 2011.

- Work experience
- PA school rotations
- Certifications
- Extracurricular activities (optional)

If you are creating a resume using a template from the internet or a word processing program, it is likely that you will follow the format suggested. While templates are a great way to organize all of your information, keep in mind that not all formats are appropriate for healthcare use (many of the templates were created for business professionals). I would encourage you to avoid including the "Objective" section in your resume. Anyone reviewing your resume recognizes that you are a PA seeking employment—you do not need to restate the obvious. Besides, you will already be sending along a cover letter providing more details about your skills and interests and how they apply to the job you are seeking.

When advising my students (and some of my colleagues), I have seen many resumes that are riddled with grammatical and content errors. One mistake new grads often make is that they include non-pertinent work information on their resume. For example, a new grad may put his or her work experience at a local fast food restaurant or a babysitting job on the resume. Unless this is extremely relevant to your professional career, it should be omitted from your professional CV or resume. However, if you worked in a healthcare setting before becoming a physician assistant, this is definitely relevant.

As a new grad, you should be able to get some help with your CV or resume from your PA program. Ask a faculty member to take a look at your resume. They are often happy to do this, and many of them consider it part of their job.

There are also PA organizations that will offer to help you with your resume. For example, AASPA offers a free resume critique service for new PAs. To take them up on this, visit their website at: http://www. aaspa.com. The AAPA also offers information about creating resumes and cover letters. They do not directly offer resume review, but they do sell books on their website that are geared for assisting new graduates with securing a job. By now, you should know that the AAPA website is: http://www.aapa.org.

To get the best help, make sure you proofread your resume before sending it on—to jobs, or even those people you are asking for help. Your reviewers should be reviewing your resume for "nits"—not reformatting or respelling it wholesale. I cannot emphasize the personal proofreading step enough! Print it out and read it aloud—this will help you find mistakes as well. Also, make sure you have used consistency in formatting. If you have used italics, bold, bullets, or headers—pick only one or two, and then make sure your use of them is consistent throughout the document. Additionally, make sure your cover letter and resume are directed to the specific job in which you are applying. It would be unfortunate to send along a cover letter that highlights your interest and experience in cardiovascular surgery when you are applying for a job in neurology. Instead of writing a generic cover letter, take the time to actually address it to the contact person listed for the job opportunity, and use that opportunity to confirm that the substance of the letter is appropriate.

On the next page I have included a template for your first resume. Please feel free to use it as a guide for creating your first resume.

Your Name, PA-C

Your Mailing Address   Your Phone Number
                                             Your E-mail Address

EDUCATION

- Public University Physician Assistant Program, Public City, NY
  Master of Science in Physician Assistant Studies, May 2012
- Anytown University, Anytown, MA
  Bachelor of Science in Biology, May 2007

PHYSICIAN ASSISTANT PROGRAM CLINICAL EXPERIENCE

Primary Care, Community Health Center, New York, NY
Family Practice, Doctor Allen Smith's Office, New York, NY
Internal Medicine, New York Hospital, New York, NY
Internal Medicine, New York Hospital, New York, NY
Pediatrics, Doctor Gloria Brown's Office, Danbury, CT
Obstetrics and Gynecology, New York Hospital, New York, NY
Psychiatry, New York Hospital, New York, NY
Geriatrics, Public Nursing Home, New York, NY
General Surgery, New York Hospital, New York, NY
Emergency Medicine, New York Hospital, New York, NY
Elective: Neurosurgery, New York Hospital, New York, NY

CERTIFICATIONS

New York State Licensed Physician Assistant, Office of the Professions
New York State Education Department, July 2012
Physician Assistant-Certified, National Commission for the Certification of
Physician Assistants, June 2012
Advanced Cardiac Life Support, American Heart Association, May 2012
Basic Cardiac Life Support, American Heart Association, May 2012

PROFESSIONAL ACTIVITIES

New York State Society of Physician Assistants, Student Member
American Academy of Physician Assistants, Student Member

PRIOR HEALTHCARE EXPERIENCE

Certified Nursing Assistant, 2007-2009, New York Health Department, NY

LANGUAGES

Mandarin (fluent)

REFERENCES

Available upon request

Using the Internet to Apply for Jobs

We live in the information age, and you will be sending your job application information through cyberspace. While it may make applying for jobs easier, it also opens the doors for casual mistakes. When sending your resume and cover letter in an e-mail format, be sure the e-mail message you have written is appropriate and without errors. As always, spell-check anything you send electronically, and check for and provide the potential employer with their requested format of your documents (e.g., Microsoft Word, PDF, etc.). Below is an example of an e-mail message to use when you are sending your resume and cover letter as attached documents.

> Dear Mr. Smith,
>
> I am attaching my cover letter and resume, to apply for the dermatology physician assistant position at New York Hospital (Reference # 002.1845). The documents are in PDF format; please let me know if you have any problems opening them or need anything additional.
>
> Very truly yours,
> Your name, PA-C
> Your address
> Your e-mail address
> Your phone number

Keep in mind that some institutions will require you to insert your cover letter and resume directly into their specific recruiting program online. You may find that your resume looks much different when copied and pasted into their software. This is because their software may not support some of the formatting that you may have used when creating your resume (e.g., bullets, italics, etc.).

While your resume may look perfect in Microsoft Word, it may look unrecognizable in the recruiter's program. Aside from making sure the information is readable and easy to follow, there is not much you can do to make it look more organized. Simply delete any symbols that show up incorrectly (bullets that look like question marks, etc.), and move on.

And, when it comes to professional e-mail, it is and should look professional. It is not a text to your niece or nephew, it should not use shorthand or emoticons, and it should not use backgrounds or unnecessary signature blocks. As we discus elsewhere in this book, you should have a professional e-mail address as well—and for consistency, make sure the e-mail account you use to forward your cover letter and resume is the same e-mail address listed on your resume.

Salaries

Obviously, salary is one of the most important parts of a job! According to the most recent AAPA census information, the average *new grad* salary is $78,405. This is the national average, so it will vary by geographic location and by specialty. Before you begin interviewing, you must determine the salary range you expect, and what you absolutely need to make the position work.

Negotiating for a higher salary than what is offered can be tough as a new graduate. If you are taking a job at a hospital, it is almost impossible to bargain because hospitals usually have a lock-step payscale that only increases based on experience. However, if you are working in a private practice, you may be able to negotiate for what-ever you think you are worth.

As I write this, if I were a new graduate, I would aim for a full-time job (40 hours or more) that offered a salary of at least $75,000 per year. If someone offers you less than that for a full-time PA position, you should try to negotiate. According to current figures, you are worth at least that much! If your prospective (or current) employer is intractable, you could share the national and state averages for PA salaries as part of your discussions. You can get this information online at the Advance PA Magazine website: http://physician-assistant.advanceweb .com, or through the AAPA where you can purchase a customized salary report at: http://www.aapa.org/research/ data_and_statistics.aspx.

Interviewing for your First Job

Interviewing for your first job as a physician assistant can be stressful. Most schools offer general assistance with resumes and interviews, but they may not cover specific details. As you prepare to answer the personal questions that will come up during the interview, you should also start determining what personal questions *you* will ask during the interview. Investigate the job opportunity a little further. Try to find out if the hospital or practice has a good reputation, if it is financially stable, if people like working there, and if patients generally have good things to say about the primary physician you will be working with. Finding out these details beforehand will help you get a better sense of what to expect and what you might want to ask about during your interview.

When you go to your interviews, take along a folder (think a professional interview folder, not your Robert Pattison "Twilight" special edition folder) and a notepad and pen, as well as copies of your resume, CV, and the cover letter you sent along to apply for the position. If you are asked questions about your resume, CV or cover letter, you will be able to refer to your own copy (rather than ask to see what you wrote). When you ask questions, or answer them, take a moment to jot down the responses. When introduced to individuals, write down their names and positions at the earliest opportunity. Also ask for business cards if they are available. This will save you time and effort when you follow-up with the employer after the interview.

To prepare for the interview, you should begin by actively thinking about your skills and interests. Take some time to come up with some truthful answers to these commonly asked questions:

- Why do you want to work in this setting or this particular practice?
- What can you offer the hospital/practice (skills, research interests, etc.)?
- What are your strengths?
- What are your weaknesses? ("I work too hard" is probably not your best response)
- Why are there gaps in your education and/or work experiences?

- Why did you leave your last job?
- What are your long-term goals?

Practicing these answers out loud will allow you to be more confident when you are actually on the interview, and may help combat any nervousness. You can also jot down some notes on your responses on the notepad you will take to the interview, so you do not forget an important point.

In addition to being prepared to answer the questions, you should also be prepared to ask your own questions about the job and the setting. Think about what information you will need to know in order to make a decision about the position. It is a good idea to write down your questions before you go to the interview and bring them along, so you can write in the answers while you are there. Consider asking the following:

- What will my role be in this setting?
- Have you ever had a physician assistant work here before? If so, how long did they stay and why did they leave?
- What will my responsibilities be outside of patient care?
- What is a typical work day like?
- What hours will I be expected to work each day and week?
- Will the job require me to work weekends, holidays, or to be on-call?
- Will I work in one hospital/clinic or will I be working at satellite offices?
- Will there be an opportunity for professional growth?
- What procedures will I be expected to do?
- Are there any procedures I will not be allowed to do?
- How many patients will I be expected to see each day?
- Will I be supervising any other staff?
- Will I have specific billing responsibilities?
- Will I be seeing patients with you (the physician), or separately?

When you begin the actual interview, be sure you are dressed appropriately. You should wear a suit and appear well groomed (this is true for both sexes). Greet the interviewer with a firm handshake and try to maintain eye contact throughout the interview. Be aware of what your body language might suggest during the interview as you want to convey confidence, competence, and friendliness.

It is a good idea to observe the setting as you walk through the hospital or office. Is it clean and welcoming? Do you feel comfortable in the environment? Does it appear safe? Does the staff appear pleasant? Do the charts or filing areas appear organized? Do the physician assistants have offices—and are they shared or separate? Most importantly, could you see yourself working there?

During the interview, you may run into a question that you are not sure how to answer. If that happens, be polite and simply tell the interviewer that you are not sure. Be honest! The interviewer knows you are a new graduate; therefore, he should not expect you to know everything.

Some interviewers will not bring up salary on the first interview and may decide to wait until offering you the position before discussing money issues. However, if it does come up, be prepared to ask about the salary range, malpractice insurance, and benefits and have that question list with you for your notes as well.

When discussing salary, make sure you ask the following questions— these will help you make your decision about the position, or to compare and contrast different opportunities.
- What is the salary range?
- Who pays malpractice insurance and what does it cover?
- Are there any bonuses or incentives?
- What are the healthcare benefits? Do they include vision, dental, life, and disability?
- How much time is offered for continuing medical education?
- How much financial support is offered for continue medical education activities?
- How much time is allowed for vacation, sick leave, and maternity leave (if applicable)?
- What are the retirement plans – is there a 401(k) or 403(b) program (with or without matching?), or a pension plan?

Before the end of your interview, try to meet all members of the team or practice that you will be working with. (In a hospital setting this may be difficult). Remember when you are working full-time as a PA, you will be spending a lot of time with these people, so it is wise to get a feel as to whether you will be able to get along with each of them.

At the end of the interview, make sure you establish clear communication regarding follow up. Will you contact them if you are interested, or will they contact you? After your interview, follow-up with a *handwritten* thank you note regardless of your decision—even if have decided you are not interested in the position. For your reference, I have included two example thank you notes below.

Interested in Job

Dr. Doe (and staff),

Thank you for inviting me to interview at your place of employment earlier this week. I appreciate you taking the time out of your busy day to show me around the office and to introduce me to the staff. I was especially impressed by the spacious patient exam rooms, and the friendliness of the staff—and enjoyed speaking with [**insert names**]. I look forward to hearing more about the PA job opportunity and whether or not I might be selected, once you have completed your interviews.

Thank you again,
Bob Smith, PA-C

Not Interested in Job

Dr. Doe (and staff),

Thank you for allowing me to interview at your place of employment earlier this week. I appreciate you taking the time out of your busy day to show me around the hospital and to introduce me to the staff. While I enjoyed meeting you, I do not feel as though this opportunity would be a good fit for me as I begin my career as a physician assistant. Once again, I thank you for the opportunity to interview, and I wish you the best of luck in finding an appropriate candidate for the position.

Thank you,
Bob Smith, PA-C

Telephone or Video Conference Interviews

While the telephone or video conference formats are not normal for most PA interviews, if you have applied for position that is not within driving distance, this type of interview may be arranged. Many hospitals and private practices have tight budgets, so an electronic interview is a convenient way to conduct the first (and sometimes only) interview. Of course, this initial conversation is usually followed by an in-person interview when both you and the physician or hospital can make arrangements for you to visit. As with every step of your application process, before you set up a phone interview, make sure that your voicemail message is professional and appropriate.

When scheduling such an interview, be sure to think hard about where you will be and what the environment will be like around you. Ideally, you would like to be sitting at home in front of a desk or computer, by yourself. If you set the interview up while you have children over, or the television or radio is playing in the background, this can be distracting and can even sabotage your likelihood of obtaining the job. Carefully examine your schedule before agreeing to a teleconference to make sure that the interview conditions are as ideal as possible. Additionally, make sure you are dressed appropriately for a video interview.

When conducting the interview, try to use a land-line or reliable internet source if you can. Cell phones occasionally lose their signal, and this would certainly make the interview more challenging. Also, avoid putting the potential employer on speakerphone; this can add echoes or static to the conversation, making it difficult for both parties to understand one another—and might even lead to a misunderstanding about the job! You may want to invest in a headset to use during a phone or internet interview if you have concerns about communicating clearly.

Substantively, prepare for telephone or internet interviews in the same way you would for an in-person interview—good habits are important. Have your resume, pen and paper, and your datebook or calendar set-up right next to you before the call begins. Because the interview may not actually be able to see your interest and enthusiasm in-person, try to sound energetic and engaged in the conversation—and avoid disinterest or obvious distraction. Do not turn on your web browser before or during the call!

The interview will likely be shorter than an in-person interview, and may range anywhere from 15-30 minutes, depending on how many people you are interviewing with. When you have completed the interview, thank whoever conducted the interview and ask what the next step in the process will be.

Once you have finished the interview, remember to send a thank you note just as you would in an in-person interview.

Receiving a Job Offer

Many times when you receive a job offer, you will receive an "offer letter." The offer letter simply states that the institution or physician has decided to offer you the job. The offer letter will often mention the salary, the healthcare benefits, the retirement plan, and a date that you must respond by in order to accept the offer. Not all employers will provide an offer letter, or a "professional" one; this is especially true in private practice settings with limited staffing.

Once you have received a job offer, review the letter and confirm it covers everything you need to know. If it does not, be sure to ask the potential employer to provide you with the information you need. I have made a list below of some of the items you will want to see in writing in the offer letter:

- Clarification as to whether the position is full-time, part-time, per-Diem, or contract work
- Expected work hours per day or week
- If there is a probation period (and if so, how long does it last?)
- Salary or hourly wage (including overtime, on-call, and night shift or weekend shift differential)
- Vacation/Holiday time
- Sick time
- Retirement plan options
- CME time and CME reimbursement
- Credentialing support

- Health insurance
- Opportunities for bonus pay or raises

After carefully reviewing the information, decide whether or not to accept the offer. If you accept, congratulations! But, if you do not feel good about the opportunity, let me assure you that it is perfectly acceptable to politely decline—this is a business decision for both parties, and you should not feel personally responsible for a practice's success just because you interviewed there. Be sure to send a letter informing the potential employer of your decision, thank them for the opportunity, and begin your search again. You will find a job that is a good fit; it just may not be the first opportunity you consider.

Contract Negotiations

If you decide to work for a private physician, it is likely you will have to create a contract. Some physicians may suggest an oral contract, but I strongly advise against this. (Even though Dr. Smith seems nice enough and encourages you to just "shake on it," this is simply not a good idea—for either party!) You never know what will happen in the future, so it is wise to create a contract that you both agree upon and both sign. This will, if nothing else, give you peace of mind if a disagreement or conflict arises at a later date. It is also advisable to have an attorney review the contract, especially if you do not understand parts of it.

Below is an example of a generic contract, and not necessarily a comprehensive one. You may encounter something similar when you begin to negotiate salary or benefits. In this section, I will cover what the generic contract does—and does not—properly outline. This is provided only for your review, and does not represent legal advice or something you should rely on. You absolutely should consult an attorney directly if you have any questions.

Dear Employee:

I am pleased to offer you a job at the office of John Smith, M.D. This letter confirms our understanding of the terms and conditions of your offer of employment. Please read and sign this letter if you agree with the details. If there are any questions or you need clarification, please let me know so we can resolve them as soon as possible.

The terms of your employment are as follows:

Position: Physician Assistant

Hours: 7:15 a.m. – 5:30 p.m. Monday through Friday. No extra pay for overtime.

Salary: $80,000 per annum, before taxes. Salary checks are issued every other week.

Start Date: July 1, 2012

Term: The term of this agreement is for one (1) year. It is our intent that this arrangement be a long-term one that is reviewed and amended annually based on your performance and productivity. However, your employment may be terminated immediately "for cause," including, but not limited to, death, disability, loss of professional licensure, or your failure to perform your duties in accordance with the high professional standards of my office, such determination to be made solely within my discretion. However, during the probation period (as hereinafter defined) your employment may be terminated at any time, effective immediately. After the probationary period, your employment may also be terminated by either party "without cause" upon sixty (60) days written notice. Unless specifically terminated in writing with proper notice, this contract will automatically renew from year-to-year after the expiry date, until further notice, under the terms and conditions described herein. In the event that this contract is automatically renewed and new terms are agreed after the expiry date, those new terms will be applied retroactively to the date of the automatic renewal.

Dues, License, Books, Journals, and CME: For the account of the practice, not to exceed $2,000.

Malpractice Insurance: For the account of the practice, for limits of $1,000,000/$3,000,000.

Non-compete Agreement: None, if going to a non-competing specialty, or if employment terminates within the first three (3) months during the probationary period. Non-compete extends to five (5) miles of our office if moving to a competing practice. The non-compete contract will extend for up to two (2) years from the time of departure at the discretion of the employer.

Probation: You will be on probation for ninety (90) days from the first date of your full time employment as a physician assistant. Your benefits will begin accruing after the first day of your full time employment.

Benefits: The following benefits apply:

Vacation and CME: You will begin to accrue three (3) weeks of vacation per year from the first date of your full time employment. Vacation accrues evenly over one (1) year.

Personal and Sick Days: You will accrue one (1) sick day per quarter, beginning after six (6) months of employment. No personal days are permitted until twelve (12) months are completed. Personal days will accrue at the rate of one (1) every six (6) months after twelve (12) months of employment. The maximum sick and personal days that can accrue during a year are two (2) and two (2) respectively. These days do not carry over or accumulate.

Health Insurance: The practice will pay 100% of your health insurance premium. Additional family members will be insured at your expense.

Pension Plan: A pension plan will be provided for all employees who have worked at the practice more than one (1) year. Details for the plan will be provided after one (1) year of employment.

Agreed and Accepted:_____

Date:_____

Components of a Good Contract
(But with a disclaimer and without giving legal advice—
when in doubt, always consult an attorney)

In the above contract, you will notice that the length of the contract is stated as one year, after which revisions can be made. Your contract should explicitly identify the start date and the duration of the contract. It should also discuss renewal or when the contract will be revised. Your contract should also discuss termination. When beginning a new job, you do not usually envision leaving—or being let go, but things may happen that cause you or your physician to end the work relationship early.

But it happens. I left my very first job after PA school within the first few weeks. I was able to do so because the contract stated there was a probationary period in which either party could terminate the contract. Some contracts will discuss terminations in terms of "without cause" or "with cause." "Without cause" means the contract may be ended by your employer at any time without reason. So, if your supervising physician decides you are not performing at the expected level, he or she can ask you to leave, if given appropriate notice. "With cause" means that the supervising physician must point to a reason why he or she is terminating your employment, and that reason must be legitimate.

There are a variety of reasons for which your employer may never fire you, including race, color, gender, religion, national origin, disabilities, genetic information, pregnancy, or veteran status; you may be a member of multiple protected classes, and there are sometimes even more possible, additional protections offered at the state level, including marital status and sexual orientation. For more specific questions about terminations, you should absolutely consider consulting an attorney.

Your contract should discuss salary or hourly rate, bonus payments, severance pay, vacation and sick time. Make sure this information is detailed very carefully, as even minor details may be important. If you are working on a salary basis, make sure your hours are clearly stated in the contract. If not, you may end up working much more than you expected without being compensated for your additional time. A good employer will allow you at least of two weeks of vacation, but a different employer might provide four weeks of vacation each year. Sick time will vary with each practice. Make sure you have at least three sick days or personal days per year. You never know when you will become ill or need a day off for personal reasons.

The contract should also identify whether the supervising physician will provide your malpractice insurance or whether or not you are required to provide your own. It is your responsibility to make sure you are appropriately covered. If your physician does not provide you with malpractice insurance, *purchase your own*. It is likely you will be able to work this into your contract because it is extremely important protection for both you and your employer.

Your contract should also have a clear job description—and you will notice that the contract above does *not* describe the position or its responsibilities.   Make sure your contract details exactly what is expected of you. A good employer with an idea of your job responsibilities should provide you with this information in writing if requested.

A good contract will also discuss fringe benefits. These usually include CME fees, licensure fees, travel expenses related to educational programs, professional organization dues, etc. Currently, industry standards suggest fringe benefits should be around $1,500-$3,000 per year. As a PA, you will have many professional fees to pay each year and they can add up surprisingly quickly. I would not sign a contract that offered less than $1,500 per year in fringe benefits related to professional fees. If your supervising physician offers you less than this, make this a negotiating point.

Some physicians may offer you an opportunity to buy into the practice at some point, either as a reward for service or in lieu of compensation. If your supervising physician presents you with this option, make sure your options are detailed clearly. And, if you decide to participate in this type of program, you should definitely have an attorney review the contract.

Many employers will also put a non-compete clause into the contract. The contract above had a non-compete clause that prohibited the PA from practicing in a given area or specialty after he or she left the practice. A normal non-compete clause may indicate a five or ten mile radius (depending on whether the location is metropolitan or rural), and may last anywhere from one to three years after you leave the job.

If an employer presents you with a contract, do not sign it right there and then. I repeat: do not sign it right away! A legitimate contract (and good job opportunity) is not a limited-time, on-the-spot offer. Take the contract home, read it through carefully, and if you can afford to have an attorney review it, you should do this as well. If there are parts of the contract you are uncomfortable with, cross them out and write in your alternative. While it may look official, a contract is only words on paper. In the end, it is what agreed to that is important.

Additionally, remember that this contract is only your initial opportunity to negotiate. If you do not believe one or more parts of the contract are fair, discuss this with your employer. Bargain for what you want, and once you are both happy with the contract feel free to sign it. And, after signing it, *always* make sure you receive a copy of it for your records. You will likely need to refer to it at a later date.

Credentialing and Privileging

As a new physician assistant, it is likely that you have little experience with credentialing or privileging. But, in order for you to work in hospitals as a physician assistant, you will have to obtain clinical privileges or credentials. The Joint Commission on Accreditation of Healthcare Organizations ("JCAHO") medical staff standards require that hospitals properly credential and privilege physician assistants. Despite the new terminology, this just means that a condition of your employment in a hospital is the verification, by the hospital, that you are a certified physician assistant or PA-C.

The hospital may start the process, or you may have to make an affirmative effort to get the process started—either way, collecting the information required to complete the process beforehand will cut down on the time you will have to wait before starting work.

To properly credential you, the hospital credentialing department will ask for a number of documents. These may include:

- Copies of your state PA license
- Proof that you have passed the PANCE (The NCCPA has recently gone paperless, so if you were never given a certificate from the NCCPA verifying your credentials, the hospital may be required to check your credentials online)
- Your DEA license (if you have one)
- National Provider Identification Number ("NPI")
- Proof of your degree from your PA program
- Proof or records of degrees from other schools or training institutions
- Proof that you have taken and passed Basic Cardiac Life Support or Advanced Cardiac Life Support
- Additional coursework specific to your new employment
- Records of any legal actions taken against you
- Proof of malpractice insurance (if they are not providing it for you)
- Letters of reference or recommendation from other clinicians that can testify to your scope of practice or level of skill

Obtaining hospital credentials or privileges is a lengthy process. Depending on your specific work setting and the type of privileges you must obtain, the process can take anywhere from one day to several months. A friend of mine had to wait nearly eight weeks in order to receive privileges in the specific hospital she was to work in. Luckily for her, she was able to start working in her supervising physician's private practice beforehand (where she did not need privileges to work). I advise you to provide your employer with all of the necessary documents for obtaining credentialing and privileging as early as possible, because you never know how long the process will take, and unless you are as lucky as my friend, that delay will delay your start day for work, and your first paycheck.

Hospitals usually define how they will grant a clinician these privileges in their medical staff bylaws. If you are curious about the specific process of your institution, or just to double check your own status, you should review those medical staff bylaws.

For further information on this topic, please review the AAPA's website at: http://www.aapa.org/your_pa_practice/practice_regulation .aspx.

What to Know Before Beginning a Job

Before working in a state, familiarize yourself with some of the state's basic laws. First, determine whether or not there are medical chart co-signature laws; if there are, determine the time frame for that co-signature that is required for compliance. Second, find out if your supervising physician needs to countersign your orders or your pre-scriptions. Some of these laws are made additionally challenging by electronic medical record systems, but hospitals and private practice sites need to find ways to comply with the laws. Every state has different laws, so this is definitely an area you need to research. Do not undertake this path alone—speak with the physicians, PAs, and other practitioners at your workplace. It is unlikely that you will be the first to ask questions (but if you are the first, be very, very cautious when determining your next steps—in that case, you should reach out further to any national or state PA organizations you belong to).

Prescribing Medications

As a practicing PA, you should have a solid understanding of what your prescription rights are. Currently, all fifty states, the District of Columbia, and Guam have given PAs prescribing rights. But each state and territory has its own, specific laws for what PAs are able to pre-scribe. Look these up, and make sure you understand your state's specific laws regarding prescription rights, especially narcotics. Research those laws, and review them. Even if no one has told you what you can and cannot do, as a licensed professional, you are ex-pected—and required—to have a firm grasp on allowed prescriptive behavior. Preparation for a deposition in a medical malpractice case (more common now for PAs than even five or ten years ago) is not the time to come "up-to-speed" on PA prescription rights in your jurisdic-tion.

Narcotics are the most heavily-regulated, prescription drugs, and the U.S. Drug Enforcement Agency ("DEA") has divided controlled substances into five different "Schedules" based on their chemical make-up.   The current official list of controlled substances can be found in section 1308 of the most recent issue of Title 21 Code of Federal Regulations ("CFR") Part 1300.[42]

Below, I review the most common, frequently prescribed drugs a PA practicing in general medicine or surgery will use. (If you work in a specialty, you may find that you use many other controlled substances as a part of your practice that are not listed here) This list will give you an idea of the different schedules and which drugs they include.

Again, each state has their own laws regarding which Schedules physician assistants are allowed to prescribe. You must review—and develop your own understanding—of your state's laws regarding prescription privileges *before* you begin working.

Schedule I
Heroin
Lysergic acid diethylamide (LSD)
Marijuana (Cannabis)

Schedule II
Amphetamine (Adderall)
Codeine (Methyl Morphine)
Cocaine
Fentanyl (Sublimaze)
Hydromorphone (Dilaudid)
Meperidine (Demerol)
Methadone (Dolophine)
Methylphenidate (Ritalin)
Morphine (MS Contin)
Oxycodone (Oxycontin)

---

[42] Drug Enforcement Agency: Controlled Substance Schedules. Available online at http://www.deadiversion.usdoj.gov/schedules/index.html. Accessed August 23, 2011.

Schedule III
Anabolic Steroids
Barbituric acid derivative (Barbiturates)
Buprenorphine (Suboxone)
Hydrocodone combination products (Lortab, Vicodin, Norco)

Schedule IV
Alprazolam (Xanax)
Clonazepam (Clonipine)
Diazepam (Valium)
Lorazepam (Ativan)
Midazolam (Versed)
Phenobarbital (Donnatal)
Zolpidem (Ambien)

Schedule V
Codeine preparations (Robitussin AC)
Diphenoxylate preparations (Lomotil)
Opium preparations (Parapectolin)
Pregabalin (Lyrica)

To review your state guidelines, you should visit: http://www.
deadiversion.usdoj.gov/drugreg/practioners.

Malpractice Concerns

As a professional, you must ensure that you are covered under some
type of malpractice insurance. Medical malpractice lawsuits are
common; without malpractice insurance you put yourself at great risk.
Physician assistants are increasingly being named in medical malpractice lawsuits—so it is important to protect yourself, because as a
dependent practitioner working under a supervising physician, you may
still be held accountable for any negligent actions you are involved
with.

If you decide to work for a hospital or private practice, it is likely that
your employer will pay for your malpractice insurance. While this is
an easy way to gain coverage, you will still have to review your policy
carefully to confirm that the policy covers you individually and appro-

priately. In addition to the policy provided by your employer (which typically lists you as a provider under a physician's name), you should consider paying for your own additional, personal policy for extra protection. If you are already covered under your work policy, it is likely that you will find additional coverage at very reasonable rates.

Indemnity and Defense

When reviewing an existing policy, or contemplating new or additional coverage, make sure you seek a policy that provides for *both* indemnity and defense. A policy that indemnifies you covers the cost of fixing an error or settling a case; a policy that covers defense costs pays for your attorney. The latter is especially important; even if you make no mistakes, attorneys often name everyone identified within a hospital or practice group in a malpractice lawsuit in order to "cover the water-front." Once named, you will need attorney representation (I do not recommend a *pro se* or "defend yourself without a lawyer" approach). Even a defense of "it's not me" requires work, and costs will add up quickly.

Tail Coverage

You should also explore "Extended Reporting Endorsement" or "tail" coverage. Tail coverage is important if you are leaving a job and want to make sure you have insurance to cover any claims that are filed after the termination of your original malpractice policy—or a condition that manifests long after the procedure or treatment that is the alleged cause of the condition.

The AAPA website has a great deal of information about malpractice insurance; for further information please check out their website at: http://www.aapa.org/advocacy-and-practice-resources/practice-resources/malpractice-insurance.

Personal Professional Liability Insurance

Even if your employer provides you with malpractice insurance, I would encourage you carry personal professional liability insurance to protect yourself. As physician assistants who have been involved in litigation will tell you, being named in a lawsuit can be one of the most psychologically—and financially—challenging times in your life, especially if you are not properly prepared for it.

There are different companies that provide malpractice insurance for physician assistants. However, as of the date of this book's publication, there is only one source of PA malpractice insurance that is endorsed by the American Academy of Physician Assistants ("AAPA")—it is provided by a company called Cotterell, Mitchell & Fifer ("CM&F"). To learn more about this insurance policy, please visit their PA-specific website at http://www.pavalue.com. Another company that is provides malpractice insurance for physician assistants is MedEdge. While I have never used their product, you should include them in your consideration of available insurance policies. MedEdge can be found online at: http://www.mededge.com.

Unfortunately, Lawsuits are a Reality

As a physician assistant, I have been involved in lawsuits—but, luckily, I have never been named in a lawsuit. I have, however, served as an expert witness in a number of cases, reviewing case fillings and plenty of deposition testimony. I have seen, first-hand, medical cases in which the outcome was very poor for the patient due to medical errors made by physician assistants, physicians, and nurses. It is never easy to deal with a poor patient outcome in general, but it is even worse if you may be at fault—in any way—for a poor outcome. Making sure you document events properly and have appropriate malpractice insurance is the best protection you have in a situation like this.

While not legal advice, I can recommend a few key issues to consider as a practicing PA that may help minimize the possibility of a lawsuit:

- **Respect the privacy of all patients, including but not limited to your own.** Just as you learned to keep medical information confidential as a student, you will have to follow these same guidelines as a practicing PA. Be sure to secure the patient's consent before releasing any private information about the patient.

- **Do not hesitate to refer a patient to a specialist.** If you refer a patient in a timely manner, you can save the patient's life, and hopefully prevent any allegations of failure to diagnose or refer.
- **Keep your practice within your legal scope of practice.** Do not provide services that you are not trained to provide. This will help you avoid accusations of fraud and improper services.
- **Discuss concerning issues with your supervising physician.** It is important to communicate regularly with your supervising physician and to notify them (in a timely manner) if you have concerns about a patient's condition and need additional assistance.

If you have legal questions, do not be afraid to consult an attorney for advice. You should also discuss any legal concerns you may have with your supervising physician, but remember that you may be personally liable. Take the time to determine your own, individual exposure. A good rule of thumb is to take anyone else's word with a grain of salt unless you have paid for the advice yourself.

Professional Organizations

I have personally found that PA professional organizations provide PAs with a great deal of benefits. Whether you have a question about licensure, prescription rights, or even a specific question about how to perform a procedure –you can often obtain this information by contacting one of the PA professional organizations. For these, and many other reasons, you should join at least one PA professional organization. (Full disclosure: I have served as a Board member for the AASPA). Consider whether you would prefer to join a national organization, a specialized organization, or even a state PA organization. Regardless of your choice, most organizations usually charge anywhere from $75-$250 for a yearly membership. And, you could always join a different organization each year if your practice interest changes and you no longer feel your membership in your current organization is beneficial.

In the index of this book, I have included a list of PA professional organizations for your review. Please refer to it when selecting an organization to join.

On a personal note, I really urge you to get involved in at least one organization. Take on a leadership role—whether small or large—and you will learn a great deal of information about the profession, running a business, and organizing CME events. Most importantly, however, you will be networking with many other professional PAs across the country. And, networking, as discussed in greater detail later in this book, will a key part of your career.

What to Know Before Beginning a New Job

When you accept your new job, it is almost guaranteed that you will be required to attend some type of employee orientation. Most employers will provide the new employee with a generic orientation program that reviews the institution's rules, as well as a more personalized clinical orientation program that provides the new employee with on-the-job training information. (If you are working for a private practice physician, there may not be a formal employee orientation).

New employee orientation may take as little as a few hours or could last an entire week. This orientation is a great way to learn more about the institution's policies and procedures. A typical orientation will cover healthcare benefits, retirement accounts, where things are located within the institution, how to identify resources that can assist you if you run into a problem in the future, and help you recognize what your responsibilities will be in complying with the standards of the institution. Some orientation programs (or portions of them) can be completed online in the privacy of your own home.

The great thing about in-person employee orientation is that you should receive pay for attending. (If you do not, you should question this). Before you start work, be sure to discuss attending employee orientation with your employer. Find out where you need to be, what time, if it is paid, and if there is a dress code.

I also encourage you to pay attention during the orientation, and to take notes, even if it is extremely uninteresting. It is likely that at some point in your future career, you will need to refer to the information you received at your employee orientation. Therefore, bring along a folder and collect all the information distributed at orientation. In the best case scenario, you will never refer to this; worst case, you will have a handy reference at your fingertips throughout the duration of your employment.

Clinical Orientation or Training

The second type of orientation you will likely receive is clinical orientation or training. The length of time you are trained will vary from institution to institution and from person to person. I received three weeks of training when I began my first hospital job as a physician assistant, but in my second job as a physician assistant, I received only one day of training. Your training period may last anywhere from one day to a few months, depending on the practice setting, type of work, and current staffing needs. Although training periods can be tedious, be sure you are comfortable with what is expected of you before agreeing to work autonomously.

During your training period, you should try to find out the following important items:

- Who to talk to if you want to take time off
- Who to talk to regarding your health insurance
- Who to talk to if you are injured at work
- Who to talk to if you have a problem with a member of the staff
- Where the cleanest bathrooms are located (seriously, this is important)
- Where the library is located (if you work in a hospital)
- What your computer passwords will be (I advise you to write these down, but keep them in a safe location!)
- Where the clean supply closet is located and if there a password or combination
- Where the best break-rooms (and cleanest refrigerators!) or call-rooms are located
- Who to talk to if you have a problem with your mobile device
- Who to talk to if you have a problem with getting paid, or if you have a question about the amount you were paid
- Who to talk to about reimbursement for CME time (and find out what paperwork is necessary)

Take advantage of the employee orientation and the training period you are given. Ask lots of questions and try to learn as much as you can. Once you are on your own, you will have much more autonomy and responsibility, so if you can figure out the basics during your training period, transitioning into solo work will be much easier. Remember, it is your responsibility to take charge of setting up your health insurance and retirement accounts. No one else will be worried about these issues, so make sure you are proactive about setting them up as early as possible.

In my first hospital job as a physician assistant, I did not realize that I would have to initiate the health insurance plan myself. I became eligible for health insurance after 90 days of employment, but it was not until my fifth month of employment that I realized I had qualified for the plan. For some reason, I assumed that someone would notify me I could apply. But, (surprise!) no one contacted me. It was my responsibility to initiate the process. Learn from my mistake!

First Day Jitters

It is very normal for you to be nervous about starting your first job as a PA. In addition to being scared, however, you should also be excited! This is what you have been waiting for—to finally work for pay! I have spoken through a lot of these types of issues with my students, and would like to share my thoughts on some of the most common first day jitters that have been brought to my attention for advice:

- Will I make a mistake?
- Will I be smart enough?
- Will I be able to find everything?
- Will the other people on staff like me?
- Will I like the job?

Will I make a mistake?
While you may want to be the perfect physician assistant, let me be the first to tell you that mistakes are inevitable. It is impossible to know how to do everything properly, especially when you are a new PA. If you take the time to think clearly, consult your supervising physician when necessary, and ask others for help when you need it—you can

decrease the likelihood of making a mistake, but you will never *elimi-nate* it. Just try your best to be responsible, and to use whatever resources are available to you when you are unsure about something. This is one situation where your best *is* absolutely good enough. Accept the fact that you probably will make a mistake, and if and when it does happen, take responsibility for your actions.

Will I be knowledgeable enough?

It is likely that your "body of information," comprised of what you learned in PA school and what you had to know in order to pass the PANCE, will provide you with enough information to get an appropriate start to your new job. No one expects you to know everything about medicine or surgery as a new PA—but they will expect you to learn quickly on the job. Pay attention to what those around you try to teach you, and reach out to others that you identify as knowledgeable. You may also ask your supervising physician to recommend a specific book or series of books for you to read before you start work to help you prepare.

Will I be able to find everything?

Knowing where to go on your first day is always a little worrisome, especially if you work in a large hospital. During your interview or orientation, try to take a tour of the facility and where exactly you will be working. If this is (or was) not possible, make sure you write down important phone numbers and bring them with you on your first day, just in case you do get lost and need to notify someone. If you do get lost in the hospital (which happens to everyone), do not be too proud to ask for help.

Will the other people on staff like me?

It is difficult to predict how well you will get along with other em-ployees, especially if you have only met them once during an interview or brief orientation. It is important to try to develop positive relation-ships with other employees because it will make your work experience much better. Try to be friendly—and helpful –right from the start. Most people will realize you are new, and will be just as interested in getting to know you as you are them. The first impression you give will last longer than you realize.

Will I like the job?

Again, determining whether or not you will like your new job is very difficult. Start your new job with a positive outlook! You chose this job for several different reasons and they chose you over everyone else they interviewed. And, if for some reason, you decide this was not the right job choice for you, you do *not* have to stay. To become a well-rounded PA, you probably should get different experiences anyway.

Job Expectations

It is likely that you will have expectations about what the job will be like. Making assumptions about your job is appropriate, but do not be upset if reality turns out much differently. I remember before I started my first hospital job as a PA, I imagined that I would respected and treated differently in the hospital because I was finally a PA-C, and no longer a physician assistant student. Because I took a job which employed many other physician assistants on several different services, this was in fact true.

I also expected that I would know a lot about my how to treat the patients on my service because I had done a rotation in my specialty in PA school. This was not true. In fact, there were several times in my first hospital job that I felt unsure about how to treat some of the patients I was taking care of—every day. The reality is that you can never predict how things will turn out, in regards to work or caring for patients.

In addition to those expectations you might have about your job, it is likely that your employer may have expectations about how you and your performance. I assume you want to make a great impression, so start off on the right foot. Contact your supervisor, whether it be a PA or MD, and find out if they have any specific job expectations for you and for your performance. They may recommend you review a specific book or attend a webinar or conference before you begin to freshen up on some of the areas of medicine you will be working in.

You will also want to find out what you will be evaluated on in the future, and what your pay scale, raise, or (if applicable) bonus will be based on. Many times, these are performance-based, so it will be useful to take a look at what you are going to be graded on. If you were taking an exam, you would want to look at the possible test topics—so prepare for your job the same way you would prepare for a test and find how you will be evaluated.

What to Bring to Work with You

Whether you have an entire office to yourself, or a small locker, you will have to think about what items you will need with you in order to perform your job. Below, I have listed some of the most important items, as well as some extra items if you have an office:

Necessary items to bring to work:
- ID Badge
- Scrub-card (if necessary; this is your access to fresh, clean hospital wear)
- Office keys
- Labcoat
- List of important work phone numbers
- Pens
- Stethoscope (even if you will not use it every day)
- Penlight
- Change of clothes (especially extra underwear and socks if you stay late and need to freshen up)
- Small travel size bag of personal items (e.g., deodorant, toothbrush, etc.)
- Lunch, snacks, and sugar-free gum or mints
- Books you will use frequently (drug reference book, etc.)
- Prescription pad (if you have one)
- Mobile devices
- Medications you take
- Money
- Lock for locker

Items to bring if you have an office:
- Diplomas, PA License, etc.
- Books for reference
- Pictures of family and/or friends

- Extra shoes to leave at work
- Umbrella to leave at work
- Snacks to leave at work
- Small plant
- Tissues

Staying Energized

Whether you work day shift, night shift, or a combination of both, staying energized at a challenging job can be difficult for anyone. Many PA jobs require long hours, which can take a toll on you both physically and mentally. It is likely you have worked long shifts when you were a PA student. Knowing how to stay energized throughout your full-time job can make the job much more enjoyable. After working day shifts, night shifts, and 26-hour shifts, I have come up with the following solutions and suggestions that worked for me:

Adequate Nutrition
As a dietitian, I have experience creating eating plans for people with all types of different jobs and lifestyles. The best advice I can give you is to eat start your day with breakfast, eat small meals throughout the day, and stay hydrated. Depending on your specific job situation, this may not always be practical—but in my experience, this is what usually helps keep people energized throughout the day.

- If you work in the operating room, eating small meals throughout the day is your best bet. It is difficult to predict when you will have time to eat your next meal because cases may run longer than expected, and that may throw off the entire operating room schedule. If may be difficult for you to sneak away for bathroom breaks during long cases, so plan your drink breaks accordingly. I advise you to pack small meals for yourself—specifically, high protein and high fiber items that will help keep you satiated through long cases. Try to stay away from eating simple sugars (like candy); they will temporarily boost your energy, but this leads to an energy dip—and possibly an increase in your appetite.

- If you work on patient floors, eating a regular lunch with a snack or two during the day will probably be your best bet. While the time of your lunch break may vary from day to day, it is likely that you will have a reasonable amount of time for eating each day. Try to eat a well-balanced lunch (protein, vegetables/fruit, and healthy fat) each day. It is likely that you will be participating in patient rounds throughout the day, so be sure to bring a snack for a quick pick-me-up either before or after your lunch break. Try hard to avoid eating candy and treats that patients or their families may generously leave at the nursing station as a way of showing their appreciation. While these snacks may provide you with a quick sugar high, they will likely make you more tired and increase your appetite shortly after.

- If you work in an office setting, eat a regular lunch with a snack during the day. While your day will be extremely busy, it will likely be more sedentary than a hospital job (although this may not always be the case!). You will likely have a scheduled lunch break each day, although the amount of time you have to eat each day may be limited by the number of patient appointments. Pack yourself a well-balanced lunch, consisting of a protein, vegetables/fruit, and healthy fat. Even if you are unable to sit down and eat your lunch all at once, you can eat parts of it throughout the day. If you have pharmaceutical representatives treating your office to lunch frequently, try to stay away from eating too many carbohydrates or desserts. These foods may make you feel tired and full, rather than energized and ready to work. And, of course, drink plenty of fluids throughout the day.

Here are some wise snack choices for staying energized throughout the day:

- Nutrition / Breakfast bar (something with low sugar, high protein, and high fiber)
- Almonds or walnuts
- Lean meat sandwich (turkey or chicken breast)
- Cheese sticks
- Yogurt (preferably Greek style, or a low sugar type)

- Low sugar energy drink
- Water (consider adding a flavor pack with B vitamins for extra energy)
- If you need caffeine (like I do!), drink it—just do not overdo it

Bottom line: Try hard to find an eating plan that works for you and your schedule. Try not to overeat, as this will likely make you feel tired. Eat small meals throughout the day, and <u>always keep gum and a small (healthy!) snackbar or package of nuts in your pocket</u>.

Adequate Sleep
Get eight hours of sleep a night...yeah, right! We may tell our patients to do just this, but we (and they) know that getting eight hours of sleep each night is just not practical for most people. Everyone requires a different amount of sleep in order to feel energized each day.

While you may be perfectly functional having had very little sleep, I do not recommend skimping on your sleep—especially when you are beginning a new job. You want to maximize your ability to think clearly. You will already doubt your skills; do not let poor sleep habits further inhibit your ability to make good decisions.

If you work a consistent day shift schedule, consider yourself lucky. It will be easy for you to create a regular sleeping pattern, even if you work long shifts. However, if you work night shifts, or swing shifts, finding a sleep schedule that works for you will be more difficult.

When I began my first hospital job as a PA, each week I worked a different shift. I had no problem adjusting my sleep schedule if I was working a week of day shifts—because this just seemed normal to me. I had much more difficulty feeling well-rested if I was working a week of night shifts. If I was working a night shift, I would try to take a nap during my lunch break, because I was usually so tired in the middle of the night. Even if I was unable to fall asleep, giving myself some time to rest always made me feel a little bit more alert for the remainder of the shift.

After my shift was over, I would oftentimes fall asleep as soon as I got home. While I tried very hard to stick to a schedule, I still found that I felt very tired even when I was awake—even if had slept for a few hours post-call. If you do work night shifts, *be consistent* with your sleeping schedule. Try to create a routine for yourself each time you come home from work, so that your body can adjust and so that you can feel energized enough to be alert at work and energized enough to enjoy your free time. You are the only one who knows how your body functions, so listen to your body and try to give it the amount of sleep that it needs.

People choose to work night shifts for many reasons. Working night shifts may pay more, they may be the only way to spend time with your family, or they may represent the only job opportunity that is available at the institution you want to work at. If you take a night shift job, remember that it will be much more difficult to create a regular sleep schedule, and it is likely that you will be tired and feel "out of whack" sometimes. Consider this when deciding whether or not to take a night shift job.

Proper Foot Care

I promise you that one of the most important decisions you will make is your investment in a good pair of shoes. Standing in the operating room, rounding on patients, and roaming the office floors will inevitably lead to tired, sore feet. After completing PA school, you may already have a personal preference when it comes to shoes. Most people I know wear tennis shoes or special orthopedic shoes. If you are looking to purchase a great (but expensive) pair of shoes, my colleagues recommend the following brands: Dansko, Sketchers (Shape-Ups), Ecco, Birkenstock, and Merrell. I recommend investing in at least one good pair of shoes for work—even if they are costly.

Now that you are working and making money, consider treating yourself to a pedicure once in a while. I typically do not spend money on spa services, but a few months into my first hospital job I decided that I needed to start taking better care of my feet so I scheduled a pedicure. I was pleasantly surprised by how wonderful it felt, and how much better my feet looked. Male or female, I highly recommend you treat yourself to a pedicure at least once or twice a year. It is well worth the money.

Schedules

When starting a new job, start off on the right foot by getting to work early each day. Even if you are only a few minutes early, you will make a good impression, and this will help develop good work habits. It may take you a week or two to find out how much time it will take you to get to and from work each day, so allow yourself extra time in the beginning. Spare yourself the embarrassment of starting a new job by showing up late, and arrive to work early.

As exciting as beginning a new job may be, planning your first vacation will be even more exciting. In order to obtain and protect the vacation time you want, there are a few key steps you must take:

- Find out who you must talk to about vacation time (and be nice to this person!)
- Find out how much vacation time you have each year (and if it expires each year, rolls over, or can be "cashed out")
- Find out when you can begin using your vacation time (some institutions do not allow vacation time until a specific period of time has passed)
- Find out what the process is for submitting a request
- Find out how early your request must be submitted
- Find out how much time you can take off at one time
- Find out how (or if) you will be paid for your time off (will it come from a "bank" of time-off hours, or does it come from somewhere else?)
- Find out if the system is the same for requesting time off for CME or sick-leave
- Find out when other employees have asked for time off—this will help you plan your vacation time, and maximize your success in taking specific days off
- Most importantly, request your time off as early as possible!

Keep in mind that sometimes (especially at hospitals) there may be "blocks" of time when employee vacations are not permitted. This may be during times when staffing is low (such as holidays), or when new interns and residents begin working in the hospital each summer. While this is disappointing and annoying, it does happen and you should find out if this is your employer's policy.

Developing Stable Work Relationships

As a physician assistant, you are a dependent practitioner, which means that you must work with a supervising physician. While the type of relationship you have with your supervising physician will vary from practice to practice and from person to person, the reality of this relationship is essential. Developing a professional rapport with your supervising physician that is positive and well-balanced will make your job much more enjoyable and it will improve the continuity of care is that is provided to your patients.

As a PA, your supervising physician is your boss, and he or she will usually determine what type of work you do and how you do it. In order to develop a good working relationship your supervising physician, you should pay attention to the type of work style that she employs. Does your supervising physician like you to see patients alone, or with her? Does your supervising physician like it when you take initiative and set things up before a procedure, or would she rather you let one of the nurses do that, and have you concentrate on paperwork instead? Does your supervising physician like to discuss her family or other outside interests with you? Pay attention, and these topics will help you shape a successful relationship with your physician.

When developing a rapport with your supervising physician, you should also consider *your* career goals within your practice setting. If you have decided that you ultimately want to be the senior PA on the service, this means that you will probably be more aggressive about staying late to finish extra work, asking for more challenging patient cases, and maybe even helping with employee scheduling. However, if you have decided that spending time with your family is more important to you than furthering your career, you will likely be content with the work you are given and will not assume any additional responsibilities at work.

As with any relationship, you may experience "ups and downs." Even if you do not agree with your supervising physician about patient care plans or how he or she interacts with patients or other physicians, do not let this interfere with your ability to perform your job. When you do not agree with your boss, respectfully explain your reason for disagreeing—outside the hearing of the patient, and other members of the staff. Ultimately, your supervising physician may not agree with you (or care what you think), but at least you took the time to state your case, and if you do it respectfully without making a scene, any repercussions from a physician who takes criticism personally should be minimized.

If your relationship creates too much tension, it may be wise to set aside some discrete time to discuss the issue or issues. You may find out that both of you were upset about something that is easily remedied. Alternatively, you may realize that the differences between the two of you are sufficient that you feel you cannot continue to work for with her—this is especially important to recognize if patient care is negatively impacted.

The relationship you create will be a balancing act between your supervising physician's personal style, and your own. Sometimes you will be in sync with one another, and sometimes you will not be. Accepting the fact that no relationship is perfect may help remind you that the relationship you do have with your boss is a satisfactory one.

If you work with other healthcare providers in addition to your supervising physician, you will have to create relationships with them as well. It is critical that you treat other healthcare professionals (and administrative staff) with at least the same respect you expect.

Mentoring

In any new job, it is especially useful to find a mentor, because, when done properly, mentoring is a fundamental part of the learning process. It is important not only in the let-me-read-your-progress-notes sense, but also in the sense of being a characterization of what it means—and what it takes—to be a competent physician assistant who strives to improve the profession and oneself. It is one of the ways that physician assistants learn, by watching their more experienced colleagues, and receiving guidance along the way.

Mentoring is also necessary because some physician assistants need to know how to interact professionally with other people and with patients. Career physician assistants do not just practice medicine or surgery—they teach, they write, and they volunteer in the community, constantly blending professional and personal interactions. As the profession is experiencing a huge period of growth, how the public perceives physician assistants will likely affect the future growth. Mentoring helps create skilled and knowledgeable physician assistants, which ultimately improves the profession, and makes everyone's job easier.

Ideally, your mentor will be another PA or physician that has experience working at your institution or practice. Your mentor will help shape your career within the institution or practice. He or she should be able to "show you the ropes" and to help you achieve some of your professional goals. Seek out someone that demonstrates competent knowledge about the practice, institution, and the profession in which you are working. Part of your mentor's responsibility is to help you understand your mistakes and to help you learn how to avoid them in the future.

A good mentor will be patient with you. Your mentor should take the time to point out why something is especially important, even for mundane tasks like filling out prescriptions or billing forms. A good mentor will be supportive. Your mentor should offer encouragement or confirmation when you have done something well. A good mentor will also encourage you to learn things on your own. He or she may tell you to review your anatomy or to review a specific procedure if you appear to be unfamiliar with it.

Your mentor should also help you learn from your mistakes. He or she should bring issues to your attention if you are not progressing appropriately. While it is not always fun to receive criticism, keep in mind that your mentor is only trying to help you to become a better clinician.

Perhaps you wonder why anyone would take this sort of time to assist you. Within the PA profession, there is an expectation that PAs will help one another, across practices and across generations. Every physician assistant has an obligation to teach, train, and lead other physician assistants—an absolute must if the profession will continue to create competent new professionals. This obligation to mentors to show you, the new physician assistant, the range of possibilities that are open to you professionally, is embedded in the profession. Whether you have an interest in writing, teaching, or working in a specialty, your mentor should encourage you to grow as a physician assistant. Take advantage of your mentor—he or she is there to help you! And, of course, once you feel comfortable in your new position, it is your turn to shoulder the responsibility to help mentor the next new employee.

Learning Along the Way

As a PA student, you probably learned a little about how to document patient charts. That was your introduction. Now that you will be a practicing physician assistant, documenting—or "charting"—will be a sizeable part of your job.

Many people forget that a medical chart is a legal document. What you write (or type) in the medical chart will be reviewed by many other people: mostly other healthcare employees, but there is a real possibility that the medical chart may eventually be used in a lawsuit. You should be very careful about what you write in the medical chart. When you document in a medical chart, you are communicating your thoughts about the patient's diagnosis, progress, or treatment plan. If someone reviews the medical chart, you want her to have no reason to question what you have written and why you wrote it. The best way to do this is to consistently follow the following basic documentation guidelines:

Documentation Guidelines

- Review other providers' progress notes and orders before writing your own
- Write legibly (if the office still uses paper charts or orders)
- Include the date and time
- Include what service you are from and/or what physician you work for
- Be concise and truthful
- Be narrow in your focus—do not include theories or suppositions about the case you have not discussed with—and gotten approval from—your supervising physician
- Sign your name (or purchase a stamp with your name and mobile number)
- Include your mobile number or office number (if not contained within your stamp)
- Do what you say you will do (if you say you will contact a physician, do it)
- Follow-up what you have ordered (if you ordered a test, follow-up to make sure it gets done)

Some of the most common documentation mistakes include: misinterpreted orders (due to poor handwriting), duplicated orders (due to failure of the provider to read what was already written), progress notes that do not properly address the patient issues, and failure of the provider to write pager or contact information. Do not make these mistakes! Luckily, the use of electronic medical records has helped cut down on some of these documentation errors.

I once received a page at the very end of my hospital shift. I quickly called the number back and spoke to the physician on the other end of the line. The physician contacted me because he wanted to inform me that he had just read a note I had written in a medical chart, and he wanted to compliment me on my legible handwriting. While I had never been contacted by another physician for that reason, I was quite happy to know that someone appreciated the fact that I made sure my handwriting was legible.

If you took the time to see the patient, take the time to write your note legibly so that others can read it. I cannot tell you how many times I have looked in a chart and been unable to identify anything that a healthcare provider has written. Because we hand-off patient care throughout our practice, communicating with others is a huge part of our jobs. Be responsible and make sure you write your orders and notes legibly so that others know what exactly you were thinking when you saw your patient.

Writing Orders

When I first began working as a PA, I had no idea how to write orders. Of course, I had read them on a daily basis as a student, but writing them seemed a bit daunting. I quickly learned the most common medications, labs, admission and discharge information, and tests that I needed to know for my job. Like me, you may be nervous about writing orders at first too, but if you watch other people, read other orders, and ask others for help—you will know what you are doing in no time.

When you begin your job training, write down those items that you think you will be ordering often (e.g., different labs and medications). That way, when you are actually working on your own, you will feel a little more confident about what to order (specifically common medication doses). Do not be afraid to look up information or ask others if you are unsure. It is *always* better to ask questions than to make a mistake and learn the hard way. For example, if you order the wrong test, you will not only cost the patient and hospital both time and money, but you will then have to order the correct test—which costs more time and money.

To ensure your orders are processed properly, always verbally review your order with the nurse taking care of the patient. This will take additional time up front, but it will ultimately save you time because the nurse will process your orders sooner if he or she knows what you need done. And, if there is any question about what exactly you have ordered and why, you can clarify with the nurse in person.

Electronic Medical Records ("EMR")

Many institutions and practices are already using electronic medical records, or are in the process of converting to these systems. If you are not used to EMR, it may seem annoying and time consuming initially.

However, it is far superior to paper charting for many reasons, including documenting. The programs allow you to access a patient's previous admissions, office visits, or test results. They also prevent you from prescribing a medication that a patient is allergic to or that interacts with another drug the patient is taking. The systems take some time to learn, but you will become comfortable with them rather quickly. Additionally, if you switch jobs at some point in the future, it is quite easy to learn a different EMR system if you have already become familiar with one.

Dictating

Some jobs require that you dictate patient encounters. When I was a physician assistant student, I observed many physicians dictating but had only practiced it once or twice on my own. However, when I was hired as a PA, I was expected to dictate regularly. This was incredibly challenging for me at first, as it is for most people. However, as with most things, the more practice you get, the easier it will become.

If you are new to dictating, there are a few things you can do to make it easier. Try to write down what you plan to say. While this is incredibly time consuming at first, if you are completely new to the process, it will help you gain confidence. Additionally, I suggest utilizing a template to help guide you. If you use a pocketbook guide with the essential components of a History and Physical Examination note or Admission Orders, you will eventually be able to dictate the entire note without writing anything down. You can also easily find these templates online.

When dictating, sit in a quiet room to avoid distractions. Take your time, and realize that you will make mistakes when you are new to the process. If you review your transcripts regularly, you can catch mistakes before they are put into the medical chart.

Dictating is easier if it is done right after you have had the patient encounter. If you wait to dictate until the end of your shift, I guarantee that you will forget pertinent information. Instead, try to set aside regular times throughout the day to step away to dictate or write orders. If you allow your dictations to pile up, it can make it much more difficult to get through and may lead to serious errors.

You will make mistakes!

As a practicing PA, you are responsible for everything you do. If you make a mistake, it is your responsibility to own up to it. If you forgot to order a test or if you overlooked an abnormal lab result, admit you made the mistake and move on. The sooner you admit you have done something wrong—and notify the proper party—the sooner you (and possibly others) can try to fix the mistake. Do not postpone notifying others if you do make a mistake—timing may be an important component of fixing even a life-threatening error. Just remember to learn from your mistakes after they have been corrected.

One of my supervising physicians used to tell me to "always do the safest thing for the patient." I have continued to use this mantra throughout my practice as a PA because it reminds me to ask for help if I have doubts about a specific medicine, procedure, or test that I am unfamiliar with. If you are unsure about whether something is safe for your patient, ask your supervising physician or PA for help. No one will be upset with you for inquiring about the appropriateness of a drug or procedure. In fact, they will be quite happy (and relieved) if you help prevent a serious error.

Understanding How to Bill for Your Services

Wherever you decide to work, billing and coding will likely be part of your job. Unfortunately, PAs do not learn much about billing and coding until they actually have to do it for the first time, on-the-job. While it is not as difficult as diagnosing and treating a patient, it can be time consuming, confusing, and it can materially affect how much money you or your practice ends up receiving for reimbursement.

If you have not already obtained a National Provider Identification Number ("NPI"), you will need to do so before you can bill for patient services. The NPI is a 10-digit identification number that you are required to have as a provider. Originally, the number was used for Medicare billing; however, many private insurance companies now require its usage. You can apply for a number online at: https://nppes.cms.hhs.gov/NPPES/Welcome.do. It is likely that your employer will assist you with this if you need help with the process.

Billing and coding errors cost providers and their practices money. To avoid costing your practice thousands of dollars, take the time to review your work with your practice or office manager to make sure you are doing it properly. Getting off on the right foot with the billing personnel will make your life much easier. If you improperly bill for services, she will constantly be on your back about it, and may even ask you to re-do your work.

Billing and coding personnel have a difficult job, working to accurately collect revenue for the practice while preventing the practice from (purposefully or accidentally) committing any fraudulent billing. In some instances, those personnel are responsible for all of the practice's billing and coding, while the actual providers do very little or nothing at all. In other situations, the billing and coding group only reviews the billing and coding the providers have done to verify that it is correct.

As a provider, there is great value to being actively involved in the billing and coding process (especially because if your name is listed on the bill—as you are responsible for its contents). By keeping in close contact with the billing and coding personnel, you will be able to verify that the services you provided are being billed properly, ultimately making both of your jobs easier. You will also learn whether or not *you* are doing things properly, or if there are improvements you can make to how you bill or code for your time and services.

It should be important to you to make sure that both you and the practice are getting reimbursed for the professional services being provided. For additional insight into the practice, ask those involved with the practice's billing and coding services if they can provide you with a billing printout of your services (and, if available, an additional comprehensive report for the service generally) every month. This will help give you a sense of how much revenue you are actually generating for the practice, and whether there is further room for your improvement.[43]

---

[43] Kent, A. How to Be Code Compliant. *PA Professional*. December 2010. Page: 38. Available at: http://paprofessional.cadmus.com/Index.aspx). Accessed on August 22, 2011.

If you have never done any billing and coding before, learning how to do it will take some time. It is likely you will make mistakes occasionally, as the process is confusing, and sometimes the codes change. However, many mistakes can be prevented if you slow down and take the extra time to review the information before you submit it.

On many occasions I have had charts returned to me because I made a billing error. Historically, my most frequent mistakes have been forgetting to sign something or forgetting to list a diagnosis. One of the hospitals I worked for had an electronic medical record system that sent e-mail notifications if I had outstanding charts that I needed to review for billing errors. This made it easier to remember to fix my errors in a timely manner, as the program continued to send me e-mails until I addressed the flagged issues.

Most clinical settings now have systems in place to help identify any billing and/or coding mishaps appropriately. To help you prepare for those issues before they come up, I have identified some billing and coding errors. Review these, and try to make an active effort to avoid these common mistakes:

The most common billing and coding errors are:
- No chief complaint listed for each visit
- Incorrect dates
- Missing signatures
- Always assigning the same level of service
- No diagnosis listed for each visit
- Not billing for all procedures performed

Although it may be difficult to catch-on to the billing and coding system at first, after a month or two, it will become habit. It certainly becomes easier when you use the same codes over and over again, and certain entries become second-nature. Again, I cannot overstate the importance of billing and coding properly: both you and your practice will suffer if you frequently make mistakes.

As a new PA, some of the billing and coding jargon may seem confusing. Below, I have listed some of the basic abbreviations[44] you should be familiar with and what they actually mean:

- **CMS:** Centers for Medicare & Medicaid Services. CMS is a Federal agency within the U.S. Department of Health and Human Services.

- **CPT:** Current Procedural Terminology. The CPT is a uniform numeric coding system that consists of descriptive terms that are used to identify medical services and procedures furnished by providers.

- **ICD-9:** International Statistical Classification of Diseases and Related Health Problems. The ICD-9 provides codes that classify diseases as well as a wide variety of signs, symptoms, abnormal findings, complaints, social circumstances and external causes of injury or disease. Every health condition can be assigned to a unique category and is given a code, up to six characters long. Such categories can include a set of similar diseases.

- **ICD-9-CM:** The International Classification of Diseases, Ninth Revision, Clinical Modification ("ICD-9-CM"). The ICD-9-CM is based on the original ICD-9 codes, and currently operates as the official system of assigning codes to diagnoses and procedures associated with hospital utilization in the United States. (These are tentatively set to be replaced by the ICD-10-CM codes in 2013).

- **ICD-10:** The International Classification of Diseases, Tenth Revision. In 1999, the ICD-10 was adopted for reporting mortality, but ICD-9-CM codes are still used for morbidity.

- **ICD-11:** The International Classification of Diseases, Eleventh Revision. The implementation of the ICD-11 is set to take place in 2014.

- **NPP:** Non-physician provider. This refers to PAs, NPs, clinical nurse specialists ("CNSs"), and certified nurse midwives

---

[44] Centers for Medicare and Medicaid Services. Available at: http://www.cms.gov/default.asp?. Accessed August 22, 2011.

("CNMs") who are permitted to bill for services under Medicare.

- **Medical Necessity:** Medical necessity is the "criterion" for, or a critical component of payment. The service provided must be medically necessary in order for Medicare to provide reimbursement.
- **E/M:** Evaluation and Management. Evaluation and management services will determine what CPT codes are used to bill. Providers select the appropriate code for the service based on the content of evaluation and management service.
- **PMS:** Preventive Medical Services. Preventive Medicine Services are for services that are considered preventative in nature (mammography, diabetes screening, etc.). They are based on age, they involve counseling and risk factor reduction, and they are not the same as a problem-oriented visit.
- **IPPE:** Initial Preventive Physical Examination. This is the initial examination for Medicare patients; it focuses on health promotion and disease detection.
- **HCPCS:** Healthcare Common Procedure Coding System Book (pronounced "hick-picks"). This coding book lists codes for durable medical equipment, procedures/professional services, drugs administered other than oral method, and other specific codes for specific circumstances. There are two levels of codes, I and II. Level I includes the CPT codes. Level II is a standardized coding system that is used primarily to identify products, supplies, and services not included in the CPT codes.
- **MPFS:** Medicare Physicians Fee Schedule. Carriers pay for a physicians services based on the Medicare physicians fee schedule.

It is also important to note that ICD-9 and ICD-10 codes are revised in April and October of every year. As a provider, it is your responsibility to make sure you are using the correct codes. For more information about billing and coding as a physician assistant, review the following websites:

- The Medicare Learning Network: Official CMS Information for Medicare Fee-For-Service Providers.

Available at: http://www.cms.gov/MLNProducts/70_APNPA.asp#TopOfPage
- The American Academy of Physician Assistants – Advocacy and Practice Resources.
Available at: http://www.aapa.org/advocacy-and-practice-resources/reimbursement

If you work in a surgical setting or perform procedures, it is likely that you will be required to obtain pre-certification of treatment for reimbursement. Typically, this requires that you provide the insurance company with an overview of the patient's medical history, the reason for the anticipated procedure, and a general description of the planned procedure. Oftentimes, pre-certification must be completed at least 5 days before the procedure in order to allow time for processing. Usually insurance companies do not require pre-certification for emergency situations. Obtaining pre-certification for treatment is a skill that is commonly learned on-the-job.

Unexpected Problems You May Encounter at Work

I have no time to eat
As discussed previously, depending on the type of work you do, finding time to successfully sit down and eat a meal may be a bit of a challenge. Think back to when you were a PA student and some of the nicer PA preceptors might tell you to "go grab a bite to eat and come back in an hour or so." Unfortunately, when you are a practicing physician assistant, you will not have someone encouraging you to take an hour "or so" for lunch.

You have chosen a career field that does not always allow for 9-5 hours; therefore, you will not always be following the standard corporate work and break schedule. In fact, while working as a physician assistant, it is likely that some days you may not have time to eat lunch at all.

Keep a snack in your labcoat pocket. You should be able to schedule a reasonable lunch break *most* days—your employer realizes you need a break each day, and she wants you to have enough time to eat. But, if you have a patient emergency—or series of them—you may only have time for a snack while you are walking down the hospital corridors.

Bottom Line: depending on your job, you may have to accept the fact that you will not always have time for a decent break at work. Always keep a snack handy in your pocket.

The other PA I work with agrees to take on work tasks, but does not follow through with them

In your first year of employment, try not to rely on anyone to complete your work. Your reputation is on the line when you are a new employee and you want to prove that you are a competent clinician and that you are capable of completing your work. If you do things yourself, you know they were completed, and that they were done properly. Relying on others is completely acceptable once you have created a solid reputation for yourself and you have deemed the person trustworthy. However, as a new employee, it is wise not to trust anyone but yourself to do your work.

Bottom Line: To avoid situations that might come back to haunt you, do the work yourself. If you allow someone else to help out, follow-up to make sure they have done the work, and have done it correctly. If you run across work that needs to be done, and it is unclear whose responsibility it is—congratulations, it is your responsibility. At least this way you can confirm that the work is done—and done well.

I do not get along with my co-workers

In every job, there will be employees that you will not like. However, remember two things: this is your own personal opinion, and it is irrelevant when it comes to work in the workplace. Not liking someone is not a good enough reason to let it affect your ability to work with him or her.

Work is no different than the rest of our lives—some people are lazy, some people do not follow the rules properly, some people gossip, and some people may even be irresponsible or incompetent practitioners. Regardless, you have little control over how someone else behaves. The only person you can control is yourself, and how you react to those bothersome people. So, do not let something as silly as an annoying coworker interfere with your ability to perform your job.

Try your hardest to learn to get along with the difficult coworker. If you find that someone is so bothersome that it impacts your work, it is still your responsibility to first try to navigate around the situation. But, you may need to discuss the issue with your superior if it continues affecting your work. As you consider escalating any employment issue, you should concurrently document the problematic behavior and issues you observe. Finally, if you have done everything you can to improve your interactions with this coworker, but you are still miserable, you may need to consider switching jobs.

Bottom Line: If you are having a personality conflict with someone, deal with it the best you can, and try hard not to let it affect your work. Your ultimate responsibility is to provide quality patient care.

The nurses are not processing my orders
Any PA who has worked in a hospital has experienced the following scenario. You see your patient, you write your progress note, you put in your orders, and you tell the nurse what orders you put in. You come back to check on the patient six hours later, only to see that none of the orders you put in the chart have been "picked up" or completed by the nurse. Not only is this incredibly annoying, it affects the quality of care the patient receives.

If this happens to you (and it will at one time or another) do not take it personally. Simply discuss it with the nurse. Find out why the orders have not been processed. It may be that the nurse was just very busy, and simply forgot about the orders or did not have time to process the orders.

In my first job, I had a problem with one specific nurse. Every time I put in patient orders I would inform the nurse of what I had ordered. And every time, a few hours later I would check to see if they had been completed and they had not. Each time this happened, I reminded the nurse nicely that I had put in some orders earlier in the day and that I needed them to be completed. Each time, the nurse eventually processed the orders. While I like following up and providing good quality care, this was becoming more of a problem as it took extra time out of my already busy workday.

Eventually, I had to speak to the nursing supervisor about the problem. I notified the nursing supervisor that I was having problems with some of the nurses picking up the orders in a timely fashion. The nursing supervisor acknowledged the problem, and said she would try to help out. After that meeting, I never had a problem again. The nurses picked up my orders quickly and efficiently, and the nurse who had given me the problem initially ended up being one of my favorite nurses to work with.

Later on, I asked the nurse why she had given me such a hard time about putting in my orders when I had just started. She said that I never took the time to introduce myself to her, and that really bothered her. While this is obviously an individual reaction, it is important to take note of how my actions affected this nurse, without my knowledge. It is likely that I just walked in, saw the patient, wrote my notes and orders, looked at the dry erase board to see who the nurse was, found the nurse and informed her of my orders.

In retrospect, a more successful strategy would have been to take the time to introduce myself to the nurse before just rattling off orders I want him or her to process. Perhaps the nurse should have taken the initiative to introduce herself, or restrained herself from her passive-aggressive behavior—but your success is built on your solutions to whatever you are dealing with. Sadly, your success should not (and cannot) rely on others "doing the right thing."

Bottom Line: Take the time to introduce yourself to the nurses when you begin working. Treat the nurses—and everyone you work with— like you work *with* them, not that they work *for* you. But, do not live your work life demanding the same treatment. Be courteous when discussing orders with the nurses because they want to be treated with respect just like you do. And, I encourage you to always follow-up your orders because if the orders do not get processed for some reason, it is likely you will be held responsible and no one else.

I want to use the internet at work, but do not want to get in trouble
Nearly all of us like to search the internet when we have downtime. Whether you like to check your e-mail, read your horoscope, shop for clothes, or plan your next vacation—you are not alone! However, is searching the internet ever appropriate at work?

A friend of mine had already made the decision that he was going to leave his hospital job as a PA, although he had not informed anyone at his current job of his decision. During a break at work, he was using the office computer to search the internet for a new job as a PA. His pager went off mid-break, and he had to leave to go to the operating room quickly. He accidentally left the job website on the office computer, open for anyone else to view.

While nothing bad happened in this situation, my friend was lucky even though he was irresponsible about his internet use at work. I suppose if you were going to be irresponsible about something, it is better for it to be the way you use the internet than the way you treat your patients.

Regarding e-mail etiquette, be careful about what type of e-mails you send if you are using an e-mail account through your employer. Sometimes items that are meant to be silly jokes get sent to the wrong people, and this can be both embarrassing and damaging. Try not to use e-mail for anything other than work-related or routine communications with others at your place of employment.

Before sending out an e-mail from your work account, ask yourself if this is something that you would feel comfortable having anyone in the office or hospital review. If friends or family send you e-mail containing questionable content, ask them to send it to your personal e-mail account instead. If you are applying for a different job, avoid using your current employer's e-mail system and instead use your own personal e-mail account. Additionally, if you are able, try to apply for new jobs while at home and not while you are using a work computer.

In the age of smart phones, it is likely that you use your phone for a great deal of your internet activities. I would encourage you to try to limit your phone use to work-related issues while you are actually working in patient areas. If you are on break or are outside of the normal patient areas, than feel free to do whatever you want to on your phone. If you use programs on your smart phone to help you diagnose and treat your patients, be aware of how much time you are spending on your phone as you do not want to get behind on your workload.

Bottom Line: If you want to use the internet for personal use while at work, ask when this is allowed, and where you can do this. Use your work e-mail wisely. When you are finished with your internet use, get in the habit of logging out of the system and clearing the computer's memory so that others cannot view what you were doing. If you do decide to use your phone to assist you with your job, make sure it is not taking away time from your patients.

My pager is going off when I am at home, and am not technically on the job
This happened to me often at my first job as a PA. If my pager went off on a day I was not working, I would quickly return the page and try to offer my help. Then, after a few months of getting paged in the middle of the night for patients that were not even on my service, I decided to talk to my superiors about it. They simply told me to turn my pager off when I am not working. They explained to me that my job was designed to be in-hospital only, so that when I left the hospital, I was not supposed to be on-call. Once I left the hospital, answering my pager was not my responsibility.

Bottom line: If you run into this problem, talk to your superiors to clarify your responsibilities. You should be able to reach a solution together. If your job requires you to be on-call when you are at home, you should clarify this before taking the position.

I cannot get my work done because I am constantly being paged
Once you have proven yourself to be a competent, hard-working physician assistant, nurses and physicians alike will want you to take care of all of their patients. This means that those nurses and physicians will page you throughout the day to ask you for help. While this may be flattering initially, it may end up interfering with your ability to complete your primary job. If you are constantly being paged, it can be difficult to get work done.

If this is becomes a problem, immediately talk to your supervisors. Explain to them how the number of times you are paged throughout the day seems to disrupt your ability to finish your work. Consider suggesting a system where you are only contacted if the patient is clearly on your service and is under your care. You may have to reinforce this policy with the floor nurses and other physicians. If it continues to be a problem, maybe it is an indication that your employer needs to hire an additional physician assistant to help cover the patient workload.

Bottom line: If you are being paged so frequently that you unable to finish your work and it is affecting patient care, you need to discuss this with your supervisor. There are solutions to this problem, but it may mean a compromise on both sides.

I am working with a physician who has never had a PA before—and it shows
As the PA profession continues to grow, more and more physicians are hiring PAs. Unfortunately, some of these physicians have never worked with a PA before, and they may not understand what your role can be in their practice. Sometimes this means that you must create practice guidelines and job responsibilities as you go, which is not always so easy. If you visit the AAPA website, they have some information online about working with a physician who has never had a PA before.

PAs dealing with this type of situations indicate that work relationships between physicians and physician assistants work better if the communication lines are open. In some instances, the physician may underestimate the PA's abilities, and the PA may have to explain or demonstrate that she is capable of completing specific tasks. For example, if you are working in a family practice setting, the physician may not realize that you can perform many procedures in the office.

You may have to demonstrate your abilities before the physician will allow you to perform these types of tasks. In other instances, the opposite may be true. The physician may delegate jobs to you that you have never been fully trained to do. In either case, actively discussing these issues will lead to a better work environment for both you and your supervising physician.

Bottom Line: If your supervising physician has never had a PA before, make sure they understand what value you can bring to the practice. Take the initiative to create a scope of practice and outline your job responsibilities—and put these in writing before you start working. You can always update or change them as you go.   Additionally, review the information on the AAPA website and share it with your supervising physician.

I am having a hard time dealing with the death of a patient

Although many healthcare practitioners act as though serious illness and lost lives have little effect on them, this is often not the case. If you work in critical care, and take care of seriously ill patients on a daily basis, dealing with death may become quite routine. You may become desensitized towards death and dying because these issues become normal to you. But those people who work in other healthcare settings and specialties may only experience this loss once in a great while—and that novelty makes the experience much more difficult to deal with. It is perfectly normal to mourn the loss of a patient, especially if you had created a special relationship with the patient or if the loss was untimely or unexpected. Do not be afraid to talk to someone if you are having a difficult time dealing with a patient's death. If you have the opportunity, consider taking advantage of some of the grief counseling services that are offered at many hospitals.

Bottom Line: If you are having trouble moving on after a traumatic event, it is important to seek help. Whether that help be in the form of counseling, medication, or support from family or friends, it is critical to take care of yourself. If you find that the problem seems to disrupt your ability to perform your job, you may consider switching jobs.

One of the physicians I work for treats me horribly

We have all run into an unpleasant physician at some point in our careers. I remember when I was a PA student I worked with a few surgeons who treated me like I was in kindergarten. It made me feel horrible and I could not wait to finish the rotation and never see them again. When someone treats you poorly, it affects how you are able to perform your job. It is disappointing that certain people are allowed to get away with treating others badly, but sometimes it does happen.

Bottom Line: You are a professional and you deserve to be treated with respect by the physicians, nurses, and other healthcare providers you work with. While I encourage you to focus on your job and not some self-determined level of "respect" you might feel entitled to, if you are not being treated with a base level of respect, contact your supervisor and stick up for yourself. Always comport yourself professionally throughout this type of situation though, as you do not want to react to someone's childish behavior by acting inappropriately yourself. Avoid passive-aggressive strategies. And, if the problem continues despite your exhaustive efforts, consider switching jobs.

The PA who takes over for me at the end of my shift is always late
Unfortunately, there will always be someone who is consistently late. (Curiously, this same person will always make it a point to leave on-time!) Sometimes being late is unavoidable—especially if there has been an unforeseen accident or catastrophe. But if a coworker is consistently late and it affects your schedule, this is a problem worth reporting to your supervisor. Set aside a time to meet with your supervisor to discuss this issue. You should not have to discuss this with the late co-worker yourself; allow your supervisor to deal with it. If the problem does not improve, bring it up again with your supervisor.

Bottom Line: You can only control your own actions—make sure that you are on-time and not tardy. If others are consistently late, and it affects your schedule, discuss it with your supervisor who should be able to solve the problem.

My supervising physician has a really poor bedside manner
Sometimes physicians forget what it is like to be a patient, and they treat their patients poorly. But the healthcare system is based on authority and competence. If a physician is good at what he or she does, the lack of diplomacy is usually tolerated. Additionally, patients are usually a little bit helpless when they see their physician, and they quickly forget how they were treated, as long as the physician did or said something about their diagnosis or treatment plan.

Does the fact that your supervising physician treats his or her patients inappropriately reflect poorly on you? No, it does not. It may affect future business if the physician develops a bad reputation, but how the physician treats his or her patients has little to do with how you and your bedside manner.

Bottom Line: If you supervising physician is highly skilled but rude to his or her patients, this will probably be overlooked by patients and healthcare providers alike. Even though your supervising physician may have poor behavior, it should not impact your bedside manner. Whether or not you feel good about how you treat your patients is all that should matter.

I recently found out I am pregnant and I am nervous about informing my boss
The initial excitement of a pregnancy may quickly fade when you begin to think about notifying your employer, especially if you are a relatively new employee. While every employer has an obligation to allow for a maternity leave, it is not always easy for them to find coverage during your absence.

Bottom Line: Your employment status should be protected by law when it relates to maternity leave, but lies about your situation will not be tolerated. Be honest about your situation and let your employer know sooner rather than later. Do your best to assist with helping the employer find a replacement for you while you are on maternity leave.

Planning for a Healthy Financial Future

Getting the job that pays a comfortable salary is exciting. You might have dreamed about it when you decided to attend PA school, as well as outlining just how you would spend those first few paychecks. But just as you spent plenty of time planning for PA school and planning for your new job, you should also make a plan for your money that sounds different than a shopping list.

Here are some of the common payroll deductions that you may see on your first check:

Payroll Deductions:

- Federal Income Tax – This is the tax that you must pay based on your gross income, minus any proper "pre-tax" deductions you select.
- Federal Insurance Contributions Act ("FICA") – This funds the Social Security and Medicare benefits enjoyed by our nation's seniors.
- State Taxes – These vary according to the state in which you live and work.
- State Unemployment and Disability – These vary according to the state in which you live and work.
- City, Local, and/or County Taxes – These vary according to the city or county in which you live and work.

Miscellaneous Deductions:

- 401(k) or 403(b) – These are elected, pre-tax retirement contribution programs. As of 2012, you are allowed to contribute a total of $17,000 per year, and an additional $5,500 if you are over 50 years old. Some companies have "match" programs in which they actually match your contributions or a percentage of your contributions. This program was designed as an incentive program to encourage savings, with built-in benefits to participants. It is set up to benefit you. Use it.
- Health Insurance – If your employer provides a plan, it is likely that you will be responsible for paying a portion of your insurance's cost in each paycheck.
- Union Dues – If you work for a hospital that is unionized, you will pay dues to the union each pay period.
- Transit Deductions – If you work in a big city and use public transportation, you may arrange to have a specific amount of pre-tax money taken out of your check to use for your transportation costs.

Living below your Means: Why it is Important

Chances are you have student loan debt. This is unsurprising, as the cost of attending PA school is extremely high. I can tell you from personal experience that paying back student loan debt is not fun. In fact, many (if not most) PA school graduates have over six figures of student loan debt. However, if you create a plan and stick to it, you can pay back federal loans, private loans, set aside money for retirement, and have some money left over to live on.

A key concept you must grasp is this: *live below your means.* You do not need to live like this forever, but until you improve your financial position, try to live as though you are on a student budget. Eliminating debt now will allow you many benefits down the road.

When you are a new graduate, avoid purchasing a big house or a new fancy car simply because you can. These purchases can wait until you have paid down a substantial portion of your debt. What you may not realize is that your student loans can cost nearly half of your monthly salary. This does not leave a lot of room for additional monthly payments, aside from housing costs, transportation costs, and food costs.

Make a plan for your student loans. Review how much debt you have, and review the different payment plans. Most financial aid counselors will review this information before you graduate, so you may have already done this. If so, stick to your plan!

If you have not yet created a plan, consider this: it makes logical, financial sense to first pay down higher interest private loans. The sooner you can get rid of the private loans, with their higher attendant interest rates, the better. Sign up for a payment schedule that automatically transfers the money from your checking account each month. This way, you will not be penalized for missing a payment, and you may even receive a discount in your interest rate for using this system.

When you have extra money, use it to make extra payments on the high interest private loans. If you get a substantial tax refund, use it to pay down your student loans. If you receive a performance bonus from your employer, use that money to put towards your student loans. Again, I reiterate, the sooner you pay down these loans, the sooner you can start spending money on more enjoyable things.

If you are young and unattached, you may want to consider taking a job that offers loan repayment. As mentioned in previous chapters, working for the National Health Service Corp in an underserved area for a few years may allow you to pay off a substantial amount of your student loan debt. The National Guard and other branches of the United States military also offer repayment programs that are worth checking out. The time commitments for these programs generally lasts 2-3 years, which means you could be debt free in a remarkably short period of time.

Living below your means may not be how you had hoped or planned to spend your first few years out of PA school, but it can significantly benefit you in the long run. When I was a newlywed, I lived with my husband in his parent's basement for over a year. Considering both of us had graduate degrees at the time, this was not exactly what we had envisioned for ourselves. However, it had significant financial advantages for us, and by swallowing some pride, we were able to pay down the majority of our debt and save up enough money to take the vacation we had always dreamed of. (It also allowed me to get to know (and love) my in-laws much better than I would have had we not spent that time with them). In our case, living below our means really paid off.

Should you consolidate?
Evaluate your interest rate percentage. If your interest rate percentage is high, greater than 15%, you should consider consolidating your debt. Research different consolidation agencies, and find out if there is a plan that is a better deal than your current plan. If you are uncomfortable with finances or have little experience, you should also discuss this matter with a trusted friend or family member (or professional) and have them review any documents before you transfer your debt from one lender to another. Many debt repayment programs have to support their own costs, and there may be something in the fine print— something that may end up costing you more than you had thought.

Retirement

When to retire, and how you will spend your retirement are considerations you must begin thinking about even as a new graduate. As the average lifespan continues to lengthen, most people can expect to have a retirement that lasts 20 or 30 years. If you hope to live without working for 20 or 30 years, your planning must begin almost as soon as you graduate.

The age at which you retire is very much a personal decision. You cannot begin to collect Social Security retirement benefits until you are 67 years older. The age of initial collection may become even higher in the future, as retirees are living longer. (It is also important to remember that it is likely this retirement program may not even be around by the time you retire).

Most financial books will tell you that if you plan to live comfortably during your retirement, you should aim to save enough assets to provide you with approximately 70-80% of your usual income for each of your retirement years. That means that if you make $70,000 per year, and plan to live on your retirement for approximately 25 years, you would need to set aside about $1.3 million. While this might seem like an unattainable amount (especially when your balance sheet is comprised mainly of student loan debt), the power of interest and a long time horizon are your saviors. To get a better sense of how interest, savings, and long-term planning work together, I recommend using an online retirement calculator, such as the calculator available on the *Bloomberg* website.[45] Additionally, as your savings start to grow and your debt is reduced, you may want to consult a financial planner to help you create a more comprehensive plan for you and your family.

According to the numbers above, you can see that you will need to save quite a bit of money if you plan to enjoy your retirement. Although it seems very far ahead into the future, putting money away for retirement when you are fresh out of school is a good idea. It is easy to get used to not having "extra" money if you start putting it towards retirement right from the beginning, good habits last a long time (rather than later

---

[45] Bloomberg: Personal Finance Calculators. Available at: http://www.bloomberg.com/personal-finance/calculators/retirement. Accessed on August 22, 2011.

fighting against bad habits) and the sooner you start, the longer you have for compound interest to work its magic.

The first step you should take is "max out," or contribute the maximum amount, to your 401(k) or 403(b) plan. As of 2012, you are allowed to contribute a pre-tax amount total of $17,000 per year, and an additional $5,500 if you are over 50 years old. A "matching" program means that the "matcher," usually the employer, will make an equal contribution to what you put into the account or at least a percentage of what you set aside. If your hospital or company has a "match" program, you will already be taking advantage of this if you are maxing out your plan contributions. However, if you are *not* putting in enough money to achieve the match, you are leaving free money behind.

If your employer does not have a 401(k) or 401(b) plan, consider investing in an individual retirement account ("IRA"). An IRA is a personal savings plan that provides you with some income tax advantages; this type of account can be especially useful if you are working as an independent contractor. There are several different types of IRA plans available, depending on the amount of money you want to contribute. To learn more about IRAs, check out the website dedicated to all things IRA: http://www.ira.com.

Additionally, some hospitals or employers have pension plans. A pension is a monthly allotment that an employer will pay you once you have retired if you met their specific pension qualifications. If your employer offers a pension plan, find out how you can qualify. Typically, you must work for the employer for a specific number of years (for example, 5 or 10 years) in order to become eligible for the pension plan.

Do not compromise your retirement account to pay off your loans; paying into your retirement is paying yourself first, and it takes advantage of certain tax benefits. It is **just as important**—if not more so— to put money away for retirement as it is to pay off your loans. If you have to cut back, focus on the fun type of purchases, like fancy cars and vacations. You have a long and remunerative career ahead of you— you will have future opportunities to buy cars and vacations, but you will *never* again get the chance to invest money with 40 years of compounded interest ahead of it.

Professional Growth

Now that you have completed your training and are a certified physician assistant, take some time to organize all of the important documents you worked hard to obtain. Purchase a small file cabinet (one that is large enough to hold those large diplomas that your academic institutions have given you) and use it as your "professional portfolio." Take the time to organize each section. I promise that a year or two (or ten) from now, you will be very glad you did this.

Regardless of how tech savvy you are, you should purchase a portable hard drive and a personal scanner to save your data. Taking the time to scan your important documents can make your life easier in the future, especially when you are applying for jobs and need to e-mail a copy of something quickly. (It can also be helpful in the rare instance that you lose one or more of your original documents). You should scan these documents onto your computer, and then use a free back-up utility (such as Microsoft's SyncToy) to back-up your scans, as well as your documents, pictures, and whatever else you fear losing.

In your professional portfolio, create different sections and organize your documents into those sections. I have listed some recommended categories for you below, followed by an explanation of each:
- Letters of Recommendation
- Transcripts
- Diplomas
- PA and DEA Licenses (and past history of these)
- Current Certifications and Continuing Medical Education Verification (and past history of these)
- NCCPA Certification
- Continuing Medical Education Receipts for Reimbursement
- Other

Letters of Recommendation
Anytime someone writes a letter of recommendation for you, make a copy and put it in the file. You may be asked to provide letters of

recommendation on the spot. If you are organized, you will have at least a few at your fingertips. Also, these are a great inspirational resource for when you will need to write your own letters of recommendation for other working professionals—especially if you have one or two letters that you are especially fond of.

Transcripts

You might have no desire to think about PA school and the grades you obtained once you graduate; however, your employers may think otherwise, and you may need to show a copy of your transcript in order to obtain a new job. Sometimes employers will request that you order "official" transcripts for them; however, allowing them to make a copy of yours will save you time and money if they will accept it—and others may accept a scanned, e-mailed copy.

Diplomas

While some PAs are able to display their academic diplomas in their office at work, this is not the case for many PAs. If you do not have a fancy office that you can proudly display your diploma in (or some prime real estate at home), carefully put it away in your file cabinet. You will need this in the future for credentialing purposes if you switch jobs, so try to make sure to take care of it. You might also consider scanning your diploma to have easy electronic access to the information on it, including your precise graduation date.

PA and DEA License

Your state physician assistant license and your DEA license are also important documents that you will need to keep for credentialing purposes. These will also need to be renewed every 2-3 years depending on the state in which you practice. The state in which you have a PA license and the Drug Enforcement Agency will send you a reminder to renew before these licenses expire, but having them handy is a good idea in case you have moved (and forgotten to update your address) and do not receive the reminder in the mail. You should keep past licenses for the information contained within them, and as proof that you were licensed at a given point in time if you are ever involved in a lawsuit.

Certifications and CME Verification

Anytime you take a certification or training course, you should retain the paper copy in your file and scan each into your electronic documents. You will need these for credentialing purposes and for entering the information into the NCCPA website for CME credit. Also keep them handy because some certifications will need to be renewed every year or two (BCLS, ACLS, etc.). You can log your CME information online anytime (within the two-year period), but make sure you file it away as soon as you get it. I know many PAs who have lost these documents and then later had to contact the organization who provided them with the CME hours, who spent a good deal of time asking (and paying) for extra copies. File and scan them as soon as you get them, and you will avoid this problem.

NCCPA Certification

If you have a certificate from the NCCPA, file it for safe keeping. The NCCPA is now paperless, so new physician assistants will not receive an actual certificate, but rather a wallet-sized card—copy and scan this as well. Keep all of the certification information organized as you will need to renew your certification every two years, and repeat the board examination in the future.

CME Receipts for Reimbursement

If you attend a continuing medical education conference or participate in any type of CME, make a copy of all of the receipts and put it in your file. You will have to submit these receipts for reimbursement. One of my former employers actually lost all of the receipts I had submitted. Six months later when I was still waiting to be reimbursed I asked why it was taking so long—it was then that they notified me that I needed to re-submit all of my receipts. Luckily, I had filed these away and it was not a big problem. But, the same thing happened to one of my coworkers and she ended up having to contact the conference asking for a receipt, the hotel, the airline, etc. Save yourself the hassle, and keep a copy for yourself.

Other

This is for any other PA related documents you want to save. Maybe you came across a CME course you are interested in for the future.

Maybe you went to a great lecture and wanted to save the handout. This section is for whatever you want it to be.

Continuing Medical Education

In order to maintain your credentialing as a PA after certification, you are required to obtain continuing medical education ("CME") credits. Currently, the NCCPA requires every PA to obtain 100 CME credit hours every two (2) years, which can be further broken down into 50 hours of category I credits and 50 hours of category II credits. You will have to continue to read journals, attend conferences, or take certification courses to maintain your status as a PA. This is not at all unusual, as most professions require you to obtain some sort of continuing education to continue to work. Once you begin these activities, add them to the file in your professional portfolio.

You must log your activities in order to prove that you have completed your 100 hours of CME. You can log these activities directly through the NCCPA website (http://www.nccpa.net). As stated before, I recommend you keep the paper copies (or certificates) in a folder, as well as scanning them and saving it to a specific folder on a hard drive (and backing those up). The NCCPA has the right to audit you at any time, so you will have to keep copies of the documents that verify your CME credit hours. You can find out more information about CME requirements at the NCCPA website, currently online at: http://www.nccpa.net/ContinuingMedicalEducation.aspx.

Obtaining CME can be costly, but oftentimes the amount of reimbursement PAs receive from work does not cover the entire cost of a conference. Consider this: a typical CME conference registration (providing about 30+ CME hours) costs around $500 - $700 to attend. The hotel will cost anywhere from $150-$300 a night; transportation will cost about $100-$500, and your meals will likely average at least $20-$50 per day.

The costs add up quickly. I spent my entire CME budget of $1,500 on just one conference one year. This also means that you will probably end up having to pay for some of your own CME hours, unless you have a very high CME budget to begin with. Make the most of the money you spend—try to find conferences that provide you with the most "bang for your buck," providing you with the most CME hours for the lowest cost. You may also want to consider rooming with another PA in order to cut down on hotel costs or attending a state or local conference to reduce travel expenses. And anytime you come across free CME credits, take the time do them!

Certificate of Added Qualification

As of September, 2011, certified physician assistants can register for the new Certificate of Added Qualification ("CAQ"). This novel certification is offered by the NCCPA, and was created to give additional recognition to physician assistants who work in specialty areas. The CAQ provides specialized examinations in the following areas: cardiovascular and cardiothoracic surgery, emergency medicine, orthopedic surgery, nephrology, or psychiatry. These examinations can be taken in addition to the general certification exam, but are not a replacement exam. There are also many hurdles to qualifying to sit for a CAQ exam, including: current certification by the NCCPA, having a valid state license, and 2,000-4,000 hours of work experience in the specialty. PAs awarded the CAQ must also obtain additional CME hours (totaling 150 hours every two (2) years). The cost of the exam is approximately $350.

As the CAQ is a relatively new program, how much value it will contribute to one's career is unclear at this time. There have been many physician assistants arguing on both sides of specialty certifications for many years. Some physician assistants feel they want a specialty certificate to demonstrate their competence in an area, and other physician assistants feel that the entire concept takes away from the best part of being a PA: the opportunity to work in any area of medicine or surgery that one desires. If you are curious, please visit the NCCPA website for more information (http://www.nccpa.net/specialty CAQs.aspx).

Recertification

Practicing PAs need to take a recertification exam every five to six years. This exam is called the Physician Assistant National Recertifying Exam ("PANRE"). The PANRE is currently offered in only one format: the computer-based, multiple-choice test. If you would like more information about the PANRE, you can visit the NCCPA website at: http://www.nccpa.net/Panre.aspx. The website explains all of the important details and is the most up-to-date resource you can find for information on recertifying.

In 2011, the PANRE cost $350 and by the time you take the PANRE, it will undoubtedly cost more. Similar to the PANCE, you must register to take the exam through the NCCPA website, and you can register for the exam in your fifth or sixth year of practice. Once registered, you are given a testing window of approximately 180 days from the beginning of the exam time frame to the end. You can schedule your exam to be taken any time within the 180 day time frame. But know that, if you apply late in your sixth year and have less than 180 days before your certification expires, then the time frame you have to take the exam will be less than 180 days. Also, you are not allowed to take the test more than two times in both your fifth and sixth year of practice (a total of four times).

The PANRE tests the same exact information as the PANCE. However, there are now practice-focused examination options. This option was designed to better accommodate the needs of those PAs who work in medical and surgical specialties. The Practice-Focused Component examination contains 60% of the standard content; however, the remaining 40% can be directed towards questions in one of the following areas: adult medicine, surgery, or primary care.

The NCCPA has also created a self-assessment tool online for the PANRE, which costs $35 and includes 120 practice questions. There are also several great study guides out there for the PANRE exam, although, like the PANCE, most of these programs are very costly. You may want to consider using some of your old study guides from the PANCE, or sharing books or programs with coworkers to save money.

Many PAs who work in specialized areas of medicine struggle with remembering the content from other areas of medicine that they do not have daily exposure to. For example, if you work in cardiology, you may find that you have a harder time answering questions about pediatric conditions. Once you have identified an area of weakness, make sure you spend adequate time refreshing yourself on that area of medicine.

I have taken and passed the PANRE, and can tell you that recertifying is stressful. Even though you have been through the process before, the daily job of a PA is not taking tests, and taking a board exam is always nerve-wracking. But, overall, my experience with the PANRE was quite positive, and I found the testing center and the NCCPA to be very helpful in answering all of my questions about the exam before I actually took it.

In my experience, the most difficult part of the PANRE happened before I arrived at the testing center. Taking time to study for the exam was certainly the hardest part. If you are working full-time, finding the time to study can be very challenging. If you can afford to do so, I would encourage you to take a review course a month or two before you take the exam. However, if this is not an option for you, create a study plan and stick to it. Whatever you choose to do to help you prepare for the exam, commit to it 100%. You worked very hard to become a PA and you do not want to jeopardize your ability to maintain your credentials.

Just as you used a variety of study tools for the PANCE, I urge you to do the same for the PANRE so you get different formats and types of questions.

Asking for a Raise

Unlike business professionals, many healthcare employees do not receive yearly bonuses; however, raises may be awarded to employees on a yearly basis. A raise is usually based on performance, cost of living increases, or on the institution's need to stay competitive with other local employers.

If you work somewhere that utilizes a "lock-step" system (usually a hospital or a unionized institution), it will be very difficult to get a raise. The employers usually base their pay on salary grids that only allow raises for "moving up the ladder." In these situations, the only way you to increase your pay will be by staying with the company and earning seniority, or by moving up into a higher paying position.

If you do not work in a hospital or unionized institution, and you feel you deserve a raise, consider discussing it with your employer. Before doing so, review your employment manual to find out if there is a policy on asking for a raise. If there is a policy, follow the rules. If there is not a policy, then start making a case for your raise—it will be up to you to prove that you are worth the extra pay. Have you earned an additional certification or degree? Or, have you taken on extra responsibilities at work? Have you started performing more billable procedures than you did when you first began working?

Find out why *exactly* you think deserve a raise, and put it in writing. Think about how much you would like to ask for, and be realistic. Once you have done these things, talk to your employer about setting up a specific time to talk. Then you can present your case. Be prepared for the fact that your employer may say no. If you feel that you are valuable to your employer, and they are unable to pay you what you feel you deserve, you may want to consider looking for another job.

When to Move On

Deciding when to leave your current job and move on is a difficult decision. If you are unhappy at work, it is easy start thinking that the "grass is greener" elsewhere, but the reality is, of course, that nearly every job is difficult, and almost none are perfect (I have yet to hear of the perfect job, but I remain an optimist). Switching jobs is a transition that, if it does happen, usually occurs 1-3 years into one's first job. The good news: changing jobs usually leads to equal or greater pay, because you are an experienced physician assistant and no longer a new graduate. The bad news: job switches are always stressful, and even salary increases do not guarantee happiness.

On that note, I recall research that indicated that the ideal salary for happiness in the western world is $73,000, or just about what you should expect as a new PA graduate. That is, happiness increases until your salary hits that number. However, once you do hit that number, your happiness does not increase further (based on salary) and the average person then thinks that she will only be happy with a 10% increase. Remember this when you are considering your next position move, if you are switching solely on the basis of compensation.

How do you determine whether or not you should stay put, or move on? This is a difficult question to answer, because it is based on a number of reasons—most of them specific to each person and his or her individual situation.

One reason to switch jobs is simply because you are "burned out." Many physician assistants take very demanding, high stress, and high paying first jobs simply to get experience. This type of job requires that you work long day shifts, night shifts, and/or weekend shifts, doing work that is mentally and physically challenging. The job requires such a demanding work schedule that, even though the physician assistant is getting terrific experience, she eventually feels exhausted and wants to work in a less stressful job with a more consistent schedule. This is a great reason to consider switching jobs.

A good friend of mine took a very prestigious cardiothoracic surgery job right after graduating from PA school. She was immediately first assisting in the operating room, managing patients in the cardiac intensive care unit, and managing cardiac floor patients. She was on-call at the hospital nearly three nights a week, in addition to working 50+ hours each week. For a while, she really enjoyed what she was doing because she felt as though she was learning a lot and she was getting great experience. However, after a year and one-half at this job, she simply burned out and could no longer perform her job because she was exhausted.

She began looking for a different job, and because she had gotten such great experience already in her first job, she easily found a cardiotho-racic job working a much more consistent schedule, making even more money than she had at her first job. Her successful lateral career move was in large part due to the fact that she had taken on such a demanding job that allowed her to obtain the breadth of experience that she did. She had "paid her dues" with hard work, and reaped the reward of a great second opportunity.

Another reason to consider leaving your current job is if you feel as though there is no more for you to learn, or no possibility of you advancing up the ladder. Some jobs are just designed to be "starter jobs" in that they allow you to learn the basics and to get some experience. If you feel as though you need to be challenged by your job and you are not getting that at work, first discuss the issue with your supervisor. He or she may help provide you with the additional responsibility or challenge that you have requested. Or, he or she might encourage you to start looking for something new as well.

If there is an opportunity for advancement at your current job and you are interested in pursuing it, be prepared to work hard. You will need to put in a lot of time and energy to excel at your job. And job excellence is not limited to working hard at the job—you will also need to concurrently network, demonstrate leadership, and exhibit innovative thinking. You may also need to obtain further educational training in order to get the position you really want.

Another reason to leave your current job is if your dislike for your work begins to affect your ability to adequately perform your duties. This might even happen unexpectedly, for no identifiable reason. However, if you find yourself hating your job and not being able to get through the work because of it, then it is probably time to look for something new.

Remember, you do not have to switch jobs if you do not want to, even if all your friends are switching their places of employment! If you were lucky enough to find your dream job, then stay and enjoy it. This information is just to help those people who might be debating whether or not they should leave their current job.

Finally, and perhaps most importantly, as long as you are not in physical danger (or about to put someone else in physical danger) do *not* quit your job until you have a new job offer already. If you plan on continuing to work at a new job, unless you can afford to live without a paycheck for at least several months (or even longer), you should not quit your job if you do not have something else already lined up. It could take a great deal of time to interview for a new job, officially accept a new job, and acquire hospital privileges. Plan ahead so that you do not run into financial hardship.

Giving Notice

Two weeks' notice is the standard, expected, professional amount of time you must give your employer before leaving if you want to end things on a good note. However, finding a new employee to fill your spot will likely take a much longer period of time. If you like your employer, and want to be courteous, consider providing as much notice as you possibly can. This way, you may be able to aid in finding a replacement and may even be able to help train the new employee. Some resources suggest giving the same amount of advanced notice as you have vacation time. (For example, if you receive 4 weeks of vacation each year you should provide your employer with 4 weeks of notice).

Take the time to review your institution's policy on giving notice. One hospital I worked for required that I give at least four weeks of notice before leaving. So, be sure to read your contract to find out what stipulations are in place regarding giving notice.

Exit Information

When you have decided to leave your job, there are several "loose ends" you must tie up before leaving. Below I have adapted a list from the AAPA website that identifies some of the important items you should take care of before your last day:
- Notify your patients and other providers you work with or receive referrals from
- Finish all of your charting and your billing
- Notify your state licensing board if you change supervising physicians
- Notify your malpractice insurance
- Review your malpractice information and determine whether your former employer provide tail coverage until you are covered at your new job
- Review your health insurance and confirm that you are covered – if not, use COBRA

- Find out when you will receive your final paycheck and if there is a "check-out" process you will need to follow to obtain your final check
- Find out if there is a vacation or sick time payout that you can collect for any unused time, and what you need to do to document or support this claim
- Find out what will happen to your retirement benefits, and decide whether you want to keep your portfolio with old employer or roll it over to your new employer (or if you have a grace period to make that decision)
- Provide your old employer with your new address
- Ask your supervisor to allow you to make copies of any reviews or evaluations you had and file these away

Getting Letters of Recommendation

Anytime, you begin a new job, it is likely that you will need letters of recommendation from your former employer. For this reason, it is mandatory that you write down everyone's contact information from your former employer *before* you leave. It is also wise to ask some of your coworkers if they would be willing to write letters for you before you actually leave.

Save your coworkers contact information in a folder with other information pertinent to your job. When you need to contact these former coworkers and supervisors, you should be able to refer to this folder to easily contact them.

Most people will be happy to write letters of recommendation for you. Again, anytime someone writes a letter of reference for you, you should always send a hand-written thank you note afterward (and make a copy of their letter for your professional portfolio).

Updating your Resume

As you begin working, you may forget to update your resume. However, keeping your resume updated will be useful when you decide to switch jobs, or even as a reference of what you have done if you are negotiating for an increase of salary or responsibility. It will always be more difficult to remember specific promotions, certifications or other achievements you may want to list on your resume if a great deal of time has elapsed before you record them.

Try to update your resume once a year, or anytime something changes—such as a promotion or job title change. Additionally, take the time to update your resume when you have taken a certification course (even BCLS and ACLS). If you have had something published, you will also want to add the properly-cited reference to your resume.

In order to help you stay organized, consider adding a folder to your professional portfolio to include all of your employment information, including: your job description, any offer letters you have received, contact information of former employers, work manuals, and even your immunization records for employee health services.

Sometimes life will take you to a new place—perhaps across the country, or even overseas. If you are moving (or have moved), this is the time to take stock, update your resume, and get organized. Additionally, you will have to notify a number of agencies of your move and will likely have to obtain a state license in your new home state. When moving, be sure to notify the following agencies:
- NCCPA
- State licensing board
- DEA
- Your old employer (in case they need to send you tax information)
- Any organizations you are member of
- Banks
- Credit cards
- Post office
- Magazine subscriptions

Pursuing Further Education

Many PAs consider obtaining an additional degree. This is unsurprising; most PAs enjoyed learning enough to take the time to become a physician assistant in the first place. If you harbor a passion for learning as well, your options for further education are nearly limitless. While many PAs pursue further training in public health, health administration, or scientific research, you may decide to create your own path and venture into something unrelated to healthcare.

If you hope to work in PA education someday, you should research doctoral programs. If you would like to work in a different area of medicine, you may wish to consider going to medical school or pursuing a fellowship. And, who knows, you may decide that you no longer want to work in healthcare at all. Whatever you decide to do, research it completely before jumping in—just as you did when you were considering becoming a physician assistant.

Promoting yourself as a Physician Assistant

Despite the fact that our profession is over 45 years old, many people I have met people who still have no idea what a PA is. That means it is important for all of us to promote ourselves as physician assistants, and to be ambassadors for the profession. If you work in a small hospital and are the only PA, you need to work hard to make a name for future physician assistants in your hospital. If you have made a bad impression in your hospital, it is entirely possible that they will not hire another PA after you are gone.

While physician assistants receive little training in topics related to business, it is necessary to know how to "market" yourself. Marketing yourself simply means identifying what you are good at and emphasizing those skills. And emphasizing skills (certainly with clinical skills) starts with documenting your skills. For example, if you have first assisted in 50 laparoscopic cholecystectomies, keep track of them. You know how to do this case in the operating room, and can refer to specific numbers if you are asked for support for your assertion. Many physician assistants document each procedure they complete so they have a record if they ever need to refer to it in the future.

If you have documented what you have done in the past, it makes it easier to explain what you have done when you interview for future positions, and easier to market your skills. Many physicians who have never had a PA before do not realize how valuable you really are. If you can sell yourself well, you can land any job. Part of recognizing your skills is listing what you have done. Keep a brief journal or list of your pertinent tasks, and you will always remember your experiences.

Another important aspect of promoting yourself as a PA is being able to network with other healthcare professionals. These networking skills will help you throughout your career to find new opportunities for both work and further learning. Always take the time to meet people and to get their contact information by requesting a business card, an e-mail address, or telephone number. Provide others with your contact information as well. Enter the contacts you receive into a contact management program, such as Outlook or Lotus Notes. If your phone is synced to your e-mail program, you will then have those contacts at your fingertips. That way, while you may never know when a contact may come in handy, at least you will have it available and in-hand.

It is a great time to be a PA. Every year our numbers grow, our legal rights to practice improve, and although there are bound to be roadblocks ahead, the future certainly looks bright from here. I firmly believe that our profession will continue to progress, and that future PA opportunities will expand as well. With that in mind, here are my impressions of and predictions for that progression for the PA profession:

- **The profession will continue to grow in number.** There has already been significant growth within the past decade, demonstrated by the increased number of accredited PA programs. Due the predicted shortage of primary care physicians, plenty of evidence suggests an increased demand for primary care providers. Physician assistants will likely help meet these needs. Additionally, the number of hours a resident physician can work is limited, so physician assistants will be vital in helping to provide patient care in those areas where medical residents work. Because of these factors, physician assistants will continue to work in both the hospital and private practice settings, and their representation there will continue to grow. This growth will make the profession stronger and will improve the general public's knowledge and use of physician assistants.

- **The profession's focus will shift from primary care to specialty care.** More and more physician assistants are working in surgical and medical subspecialties. Salaries tend to be higher depending on the specialty choice, which is an influencing factor in PA job selection. Finally, government incentives may be needed to help fill healthcare shortages in primary care. (Morgan PA, Hooker RS. Choice of specialties among physician assistants in the United States. Health Affairs. 2010;29(5):887-892). This leads to two conclusions: first, PAs will have greater opportunities within specialty care, due to increased exposure within that field; second, PAs will be more competitive within primary care due to the projected shortages.

- **There will be an increased need for advanced degrees.** Most PA programs now provide Master's degrees, and it is likely that those that do not currently are in the process of converting to this standard. There is presently only one program (Baylor) that provides a Doctoral degree for physician assistants. While the profession as a whole will not require PAs to obtain Doctoral degrees any time in the near future (there is plenty of opposition to this), some PAs with an eye towards non-clinical employment opportunities within the profession may choose to pursue this path of higher education.

  As of 2015, all NP programs will provide their graduates with clinical Doctoral degrees, and physical therapy programs now offer Doctoral degrees to their students as well. These two prominent healthcare professions have moved forward with advancing the degree their students are awarded, so it is unlikely that the PA profession is immune to this trend. So, while it is currently not necessary to obtain a Doctoral degree to work as a clinical practitioner—and certainly not as a PA—this is the direction the clinical practitioner fields are taking. Finally, those wishing to pursue employment in academia should consider obtaining a doctoral degree of some type, as the PA degree is not the "terminal" degree for a tenure teaching job within PA schools.

- **There will be a need for specialty training.** As more and more PAs begin to work in medical or surgical specialties, the need for further specialty certification or training will increase. Certain hospitals and physicians may begin to require proof of PA competency in a certain specialty by providing documentation for course or procedure completion (many already do). In 2011, the NCCPA began providing specialty examinations for those physician assistants who desired additional certification in their specialties. While this examination is optional, and there are currently no specialty certification requirements for PAs, at some point in the future,

PAs will need these additional educational or clinical certifications for specialty practice.

- **There will be a need for universal reimbursement.** As there are going to be many changes to the U.S. Healthcare system in 2014, the future of reimbursement for mid-level providers is uncertain. While PAs have worked hard for the current policies they have regarding reimbursement, private insurance companies still have the right to deny payment for services provided by PAs and NPs based on those companies' sometimes arbitrary standards. PAs must continue to work towards universal reimbursement, which would require all private insurance companies to pay for their services.

- **Physician assistants will work globally.** While U.S.-trained PAs are currently working in the United Kingdom, Australia, the Middle East, and Canada, other countries have taken notice, and are considering adopting the use of PAs. Certainly mid-level providers generally will be employed throughout the world. A PA or NP equivalent may be named something different in a given foreign country, but the need for a viable global health work force to provide quality medical care in times of real shortages and emergencies will continue to develop increased recognition to these professions. Physician assistants are fortunate to have advanced knowledge and skills in all medical disciplines and as other parts of the world realize a need for more well-trained healthcare providers, the use of PAs abroad will continue to grow.

- **The need for competent practitioners will grow.** The Centers for Medicare and Medicaid Services has made several changes within the last few years to force providers to reduce patient errors in order to receive adequate reimbursement. The implementation of these programs will continue to push providers to provider fewer errors, thus providing higher quality patient care. Hospitals and private practices have focused efforts on decreasing patient infections, pressure ulcers, and hospital-acquired injuries in order to comply with CMS guidelines and receive adequate reimbursement for patient services.   PAs will continue to play an incredibly important role in following these guidelines, and will gain increased responsibility as cost-effective first lines of defense against patient complications that may lead to non-reimbursable medical costs.

- **Technology will continue to change the way we practice medicine.** The use of electronic medical record systems will become the standard in nearly all practice settings. The Health Information Technology for Economic and Clinical Health Act (or "HITECH Act") has already provided financial incentives for providers to use electronic health record systems.[46] It is only a matter of time before there is a national health database which allows providers to utilize medical records from various hospitals and parts of the country.

There are daily advances in diagnostic testing and treatment modalities, coupled with the development of new mobile device applications that enhance medical care for both patients and providers.   Currently, physician assistants are treating patients virtually through telehealth programs and online programs that allow patients to be diagnosed and treated without even leaving their homes. But, although life—and the practice of medicine— will become more digital around us, we must always remember to care for the patient as a human, the way we were trained to do in PA school.

---

[46] Shock, L. Meaningful Use – What Does it Mean for your Practice? PA Professional. December 2010. Page 36. Available at: http://paprofessional.cadmus.com//index.aspx?issue=01-dec-2010. Accessed on August 22, 2011.

Resources

The job of a PA can literally be life-or-death, but because it is impossible to know the answer to every question, it is important to know how to find the answers quickly. With that in mind, I highly recommend you check out some of these physician assistant resources, as they contain in-depth, useful information on further PA topics:

Recommended Medical Applications for Mobile Devices

Epocrates: The free version of this program provides current drug information. The premium (or fee-based service) includes in-depth information for hundreds of diseases and conditions. This is a great resource for one's clinical rotations (and a personal favorite of mine). Epocrates is a subscription service program, with different options for information and length of subscription—prices vary, but plan on paying a lot for the full content.

Medscape: This program is completely free! It offers in-depth information on drugs, disease and conditions, as well as different procedures, and is a must-have!

Liebermans iRadiology: A valuable tool for students, as it allows for quick review of classic radiology. This program is also free.

Medcalc: The program allows you to retrieve complicated medical formulas quickly and easily. Currently this program costs around 1-2 dollars.

Diagnosaurus Ddx: This tool allows you to come up with a differential diagnosis quickly and easily. You can enter in a suspected diagnosis, and the program will provide you others you should consider as well. Currently this program costs around 1-2 dollars.

Netters Anatomy Flashcards: This program allows you to review numerous anatomy pictures on your smartphone. Currently this program costs around 4-5 dollars.

IMurmur 2: This program allows the user to listen to actual murmurs, and the program provides information about each murmur. Currently this program costs around 5-6 dollars.

ECG Guide: The program provides hundreds of examples of electrocardiograms for you to review, as well as information to help guide you in interpreting them on your own. It is a great way to review for Advanced Cardiac Life Support ("ACLS"). Currently this program costs around 1-2 dollars.

Skyscape: A comprehensive guide with prescription drug information as well as an overview of different diseases. The free version of the program provides access to some of the content, but the program encourages you to purchase resources from its premium catalog, which include several popular medical books. Currently this program is free, but there are in-app purchases that may enhance the program.

Eponyms: This application allows you to review thousands of medical eponyms (such as Virchow's node or Rovsing's sign). The student version of this program is free, and the non-student version currently costs around 2-3 dollars. This is definitely worth the download during your clinical rotations.

Radiology 2.0: One night in the ED: This program allows you to review a series of different cases that simulate reading CT scans in the workplace. There are explanations of some of the common findings and items you should be able to recognize when reviewing CT scans. A must-have, as this program is free!

Mobile MerkMedicus: This applications offers several well-known reference books for free (Harrison's, for example), as well as drug information. This program is currently free, but you do need to register online in order to use the program properly.

Pepid: This program provides the latest clinical and drug information. This is a great product for students and practicing clinicians because it is constantly updated. There is a free version as well as a subscription based version of this program.

Dynamed: This program provides a comprehensive database of diagnostic and treatment information for common medical conditions. The program is updated frequently. The program is currently free, but you do need to register online in order to use the program properly.

Calculate by QxMD: This is a clinical calculator that allows you to input information and determine the appropriate diagnosis or treatment based on the numbers. This program is currently free.

BlackBag Medical Resources: This program offers medical news, tools and different resources for healthcare professionals, and is a great tool for keeping up to date with current medical reports. This program is currently free.

AO Surgery Reference: This program is a fantastic overview of the most common orthopedic surgical procedures performed. The program is updated frequently, and is a great way to review before stepping into the operating room. This program is currently free.

Audio Medical Spanish: This application allows you to review common medical questions and phrases as well as hear them aloud. If you work in an area with Hispanic patients, this program may be extremely useful. The free version offers limited access to the program. The premium version currently costs 5-6 dollars.

Thomson Reuters Clinical Xpert: This program allows you to view your own patients current information on your smartphone. (Note: You must have permission from your hospital in order to utilize this program). The program is currently free.

Physician Assistant Websites for Students

If you perform a quick internet search, you will discover there are plenty of resources available for you to explore on the internet. Here are just a handful of the sites I use regularly and would recommend to you.

Physician Assistant ED
Website: http:www.physicianassistanted.com
Content: The website was developed by a physician assistant educator to provide those interested in the profession (pre-PA, student, or practicing PA) with more information about all of the different programs available. The website is fantastic for comparing different PA programs as well as networking with others.

PA Shadow Online
Website: http://www.pashadowonline.com
Content: Provides pre-PA students with an opportunity to connect with practicing physician assistants for the purpose of obtaining shadowing experience.

Clinician 1
Website: http://www.clinician1.com
Content: A website developed with physician assistants and nurse practitioners in mind. The website provides an opportunity to interact with other clinicians online through various groups.

Advance Magazine for Physician Assistants
Website: http://physician-assistant.advanceweb.com
Content: Provides PAs with clinical articles, professional news and analysis, practice articles and opinions specifically tailored to PAs' needs.

NEWS-Line for Physician Assistants
Website: http://www.news-line.com/?-token.target=home&-token.profession=pa
Content: Provides professional news, informative articles and career openings.

Physician Assistant Forum
Website: http://www.physicianassistantforum.com
Content: A forum designed for Pre-PA students, PA students, and PAs in practice. A great place to ask questions and network with others interested in the profession.

Student Academy of the American Academy of Physician Assistants
Website: http://www.aapa.org/student-academy
Content: Provides current information related to being a PA student and the PA profession.

Student-Doctor Forum
Website: http://www.studentdoctor.net/
Content: A forum designed for students interested in healthcare professions.

Clinical Advisor
Website: http://www.clinicaladvisor.com
Content: A web site for mid-level providers that offers the latest information on diagnosing, treating, managing, and preventing medical conditions typically seen in the office-based primary-care setting.

Student Financial Resources

College Answer: The Planning for College Destination
Website: http://www.collegeanswer.com
Content: Offers pointers on the college admission process from preparation to getting loans. Also provides tools that enable users to analyze the affordability of schools.

Fastweb: Scholarships, Financial Aid, and Colleges
Website: http://www.fastweb.com
Content: The nation's largest, most accurate, and most frequently updated scholarship database online.

FinAid: The Smart Student Guide to Financial Aid
Website: http://www.finaid.org
Content: Provides information about financing a college education.

Free Application for Federal Student Aid
Website: http://www.fafsa.ed.gov
Content: Provides the application and necessary information to receive federal financial aid.

Recommended Reference Books

The Ultimate Guide to Getting Into Physician Assistant School, Third Edition, by Andrew J. Rodican.

So You Want to Be a Physician Assistant, by Beth Grivett, Larry Rosen and Denise Werner.

How to "Ace" the Physician Assistant Interview, by Andrew J. Rodican.

A Kernel in the Pod: The Adventures of a Midlevel Clinician in a Top-level World, by J. Michael Jones.

Med School Confidential: A Complete Guide to the Medical School Experience: By Students, for Students, by Robert H. Miller and Daniel M. Bissell.

Opportunities in Physician Assistant Careers, by Terence J. Sacks.

Physician Assistant: A Guide to Clinical Practice, Fourth Edition, by Ruth Ballweg, Darwin Brown, Edward Sullivan, and Dan Vetrosky.

Physician Assistants in American Medicine, by Roderick S. Hooker and James F. Cawley.

The Intern Blues: The Timeless Classic About the Making of a Doctor, by Robert Marion.

Authoring Patient Records: An Interactive Guide, by Michael P. Pagano.

The Preceptor's Handbook for Supervising Physician Assistants, by Randy Danielsen, Ruth Ballweg, Linda Vorvick, and Donald Sefcik.

Work 101: Learning the Ropes of the Workplace without Hanging Yourself, by Elizabeth Freedman, MBA.

Complications: A Surgeon's Notes on an Imperfect Science, by Atul Gawande.

Every Patient Tells a Story: Medical Mysteries and the Art of Diagnosis, by Lisa Sanders.

Hot Lights, Cold Steel: Life, Death and Sleepless Nights in a Surgeon's First Years, by Michael J. Collins.

Out of Practice: Fighting for Primary Care Medicine in America (The Culture and Politics of Health Care Work), by Frederick Barken.

The Immortal Life of Henrietta Lacks, by Rebecca Skloot.

My Own Country: A Doctor's Story, by Abraham Verghese.

A Life in Medicine: A Literary Anthology, by Robert Coles and Randy Testa.

The Anatomy of Hope: How People Prevail in the Face of Illness, by Jerome Groopman.

The Checklist Manifesto: How to Get Things Right, by Atul Gawande.

The Best American Medical Writing 2009, edited by Pauline Chen.

Index of Physician Assistant Programs

I have researched and gathered information on each of the 156 physician assistant programs currently accredited in the United States. Please use this information as only your first step; because PA programs can make changes at any time, you should contact each program you are interested to determine their current admission and tuition fee policies.

(Note: the information listed below was taken directly from each program's website)

Alabama

University of Alabama at Birmingham
Special focus: Surgical Care
Location: Birmingham, AL
Degree granted: Master's Degree
Phone: 205-934-3209
E-mail: AskCDS@uab.edu
Website: http://www.uab.edu/cds/academic/graduate/spa
Supplemental application: Yes, $25 fee
Number of students accepted into program each year: 40-45
Average GPA: 3.34-3.75
GRE: Yes
Length of program: 27 months
Uses CASPA: Yes
Tuition Cost: $61,613 (in-state), $128,502 (out-of-state)

University of South Alabama
Special focus: Primary Care
Location: Mobile, AL
Degree granted: Master's Degree
Phone: 251-445-9334
E-mail: pastudies@usouthal.edu
Website: http://www.southalabama.edu/alliedhealth/pa/
Supplemental application: Yes, $110 fee
Number of students accepted into program each year: 40
Average GPA: 3.0-3.5 (Minimum of 3.5 for early admission)
GRE: Yes
Length of program: 27 months
Uses CASPA: Yes
Tuition Cost: $47,070 (in-state), $83,370 (out-of-state)

Arkansas

Harding University
Special focus: General
Location: Searcy, AR
Degree granted: Master's Degree
Phone: 501-279-5642
E-mail: paprogram@harding.edu
Website: http://www.harding.edu/PAprogram/index.html
Supplemental application: Yes, $25 fee
Number of students accepted into program each year: 36
Average GPA: 3.5
GRE: Yes
Length of program: 28 months
Uses CASPA: Yes
Tuition Cost: $70,594

Arizona

Arizona School of Health Sciences
Special focus: Primary Care, with special track for Native American students
Location: Mesa, AZ
Degree granted: Master's Degree
Phone: 480-219-6000
E-mail: admissions@atsu.edu
Website: http://www.atsu.edu/ashs/programs/physician_assistant/index.htm
Supplemental application: No
Number of students accepted into program each year: 65-70
Average GPA: 3.3
GRE: No
Length of program: 26 months
Uses CASPA: Yes
Tuition Cost: $65,000

Midwestern University
Special focus: Primary Care, with specializations in research, clinical, bioethics, or health education
Location: Glendale, AZ
Degree granted: Master's Degree
Phone: 623-572-3311
E-mail: admissaz@midwestern.edu
Website:
http://www.midwestern.edu/Programs_and_Admission/AZ_Physician_Assistant_Stud ies.html
Supplemental application: No
Number of students accepted into program each year: 90
Average GPA: 3.56
GRE: Yes
Length of program: 27 months
Uses CASPA: Yes
Tuition Cost: $82,830

California

Keck School of Medicine of the University of Southern California
Special focus: Primary Care
Location: Alhambra, CA
Degree granted: Master's Degree
Phone: 626-457-4240
E-mail: uscpa@usc.edu
Website:
http://keck.usc.edu/Education/Academic_Department_and_Divisions/Physician_Assis tant_Program.aspx
Supplemental application: Yes, $50 fee
Number of students accepted into program each year: 50-55
Average GPA: 3.36
GRE: Yes
Length of program: 33 months
Uses CASPA: Yes
Tuition Cost: $134,645

Loma Linda University
Special focus: Primary Care
Location: Loma Linda, CA
Degree granted: Master's Degree
Phone: 909-558-7295
E-mail: pa@llu.edu
Website: http://www.llu.edu/allied-health/sahp/pa/index.page
Supplemental application: Yes
Number of students accepted into program each year: 30
Average GPA: 3.6
GRE: No
Length of program: 24 months
Uses CASPA: Yes
Tuition Cost: $86,000

Riverside County/Riverside Community College
Special focus: Primary Care
Location: Moreno Valley, CA
Degree granted: Certificate, or Associate's Degree option
Phone: 951-571-6166
E-mail: pa@rcc.edu
Website: http://www.rcc.edu/academicPrograms/physicianAssistant/index.cfm
Supplemental application: Yes
Number of students accepted into program each year: 30-32
Average GPA: N/A
GRE: No
Length of program: 24 months
Uses CASPA: No
Tuition Cost: $7,333 (in-state) and $23,620 (out-of-state)

Samuel Merritt College
Special focus: Primary Care
Location: Oakland, CA
Degree granted: Master's Degree
Phone: 510-869-6608
E-mail: pharrison@samuelmerritt.edu
Website: http://www.samuelmerritt.edu/physician_assistant
Supplemental application: No
Number of students accepted into program each year: 35-40
Average GPA: 3.43
GRE: No
Length of program: 27 months
Uses CASPA: Yes
Tuition: $88,913

San Joaquin Valley College
Special focus: Primary Care, with focus on providing care in rural and disadvantaged communities
Location: Visalia, CA
Degree granted: Associate's Degree, Master's Degree option
Phone: 559-651-2500 ext. 351
E-mail: admissions.pa@sjvc.edu
Website: http://www.sjvc.edu/program/Physician_Assistant/
Supplemental application: Yes
Number of students accepted into program each year: 20
Average GPA: 2.8
GRE: No
Length of program: 24 months
Uses CASPA: No
Tuition Cost: $55,890

Stanford University School of Medicine
Special focus: Primary Care
Location: Palo Alto, CA
Degree granted: Certificate, Master's Degree option available
Phone: 650-725-6959
E-mail: pcap-information@lists.stanford.edu
Website: http://pcap.stanford.edu/
Supplemental application: Yes
Number of students accepted into program each year: 50
Average GPA: 3.0-3.5
GRE: No
Length of program: 16 months
Uses CASPA: No
Tuition Cost: $34,465 (in-state), $43,465 (out-of-state)

Touro University – California College of Health Sciences
Special focus: Primary Care and Public Health
Location: Vallejo, CA
Degree granted: Master's Degree
Phone: 707-638-5200
E-mail: melanie.lim@tu.edu
Website: http://www.tu.edu/departments.php?id=42
Supplemental application: No, only sent to qualified applicants
Number of students accepted into program each year: 40-45
Average GPA: 3.14
GRE: No
Length of program: 32 months
Uses CASPA: Yes
Tuition Cost: $103,083

University of California – Davis
Special focus: Primary Care
Location: Sacramento, CA
Degree granted: Certificate
Phone: 916-734-3551
E-mail: fnppa@ucdavis.edu
Website: http://www.ucdmc.ucdavis.edu/fnppa/
Supplemental application: No, only sent to qualified applicants
Number of students accepted into program each year: 60-70
Average GPA: 3.31
GRE: No
Length of program: 24 months
Uses CASPA: Yes
Tuition Cost: $33,205 (in-state), $79,249 (out-of-state)

Western University of Health Sciences
Special focus: Primary Care
Location: Pomona, CA
Degree granted: Master's Degree
Phone: 909-469-5335
E-mail: mhaverkamp@westernu.edu or whitej@westernu.edu
Website: http://prospective.westernu.edu/physician-assistant/welcome
Supplemental application: Yes, $50
Number of students accepted into program each year: 98
Average GPA: 3.42
GRE: No
Length of program: 24 months
Uses CASPA: Yes
Tuition Cost: $69,768

Colorado

Red Rocks Community College
Special focus: Primary Care
Location: Lakewood, CO
Degree granted: Certificate, and Master's option available
Phone: 303-914-6386
E-mail: pa.program@rrcc.edu
Website: http://www.rrcc.edu/pa/
Supplemental application: Yes, $50 fee
Number of students accepted into program each year: 32
Average GPA: 3.3
GRE: No
Length of program: 25 months
Uses CASPA: Yes
Tuition Cost: $32,160 (in-state), $40,227 (out-of-state)

University of Colorado
Special focus: Primary Care, Emphasis on Pediatric Medicine
Location: Aurora, CO
Degree granted: Master's Degree
Phone: 303-315-7963
E-mail: pa-info@ucdenver.edu
Website: http://medschool.ucdenver.edu/paprogram
Supplemental application: Yes
Number of students accepted into program each year: 40-44
Average GPA: 3.8
GRE: Yes
Length of program: 36 months
Uses CASPA: Yes
Tuition Cost: $42,007 (in-state), $86,116 (out-of-state)

Connecticut

Quinnipiac University
Special focus: Primary Care
Location: Hamden, CT
Degree granted: Master's Degree
Phone: 203-582-3639
E-mail: graduate@quinnipiac.edu
Website: http://www.quinnipiac.edu/x781.xml
Supplemental application: No
Number of students accepted into program each year: 54
Average GPA: 3.4
GRE: No
Length of program: 27 months
Uses CASPA: Yes
Tuition Cost: $81,175

University of Bridgeport
Special focus: Primary Care
Location: New Haven, CT
Degree granted: Master's Degree
Phone: 203-576-4348
E-mail: pai@bridgeport.edu
Website: http://www.bridgeport.edu/academics/graduate/pa/default.aspx
Supplemental application: No
Number of students accepted into program each year: 20 students
Average GPA: 3.0
GRE: No
Length of program: 28 months
Uses CASPA: Yes
Tuition Cost: $73,625

Yale University School of Medicine
Special focus: General
Location: New Haven, CT
Degree granted: Master's Degree
Phone: 203-785-2860
E-mail: pa.program@yale.edu
Website: http://info.med.yale.edu/phyassoc/
Supplemental application: No
Number of students accepted into program each year: 36 students
Average GPA: 3.6
GRE: Yes
Length of program: 27 months
Uses CASPA: Yes
Tuition Cost: $73,055

Delaware

Arcadia University
Special focus: Primary Care
Location: Christiana, DE
Degree granted: Master's Degree, Public Health option available
Phone: 302-356-9440
E-mail: admiss@arcadia.edu
Website: http://www.arcadia.edu/academic/default.aspx?id=425
Supplemental application: No
Number of students accepted into program each year: 49
Average GPA: >3.2
GRE: Yes
Length of program: 24 months
Uses CASPA: Yes
Tuition Cost: $66,380

Florida

Barry University School of Graduate Medical Sciences
Special focus: Primary Care
Location: Miami Shores, FL, and St. Petersburg, FL
Degree granted: Master's Degree
Phone: 305-899-3130 or 1-800-319-3338
E-mail: paadmissions@mail.barry.edu
Website: http://www.barry.edu/pa/
Supplemental application: No
Number of students accepted into program each year: 52 (Miami), and 24 (St. Petersburg)
Average GPA: >3.0
GRE: Yes
Length of program: 28 months
Uses CASPA: Yes
Tuition Cost: $77,925

Miami Dade College
Special focus: Primary Care
Location: Miami, FL
Degree granted: Associate's Degree
Phone: 305-237-4160
E-mail: jhernan7@mdc.edu
Website: http://www.mdc.edu/medical/AHT/PA/default.asp
Supplemental application: Yes, $25 fee
Number of students accepted into program each year: 40
Average GPA: >2.5
GRE: No
Length of program: 24 months
Uses CASPA: No
Tuition Cost: $25,770 (in-state), $39,814 (out-of-state)

Keiser University
Special focus: Primary Care
Location: Fort Lauderdale, FL
Degree granted: Master's Degree
Phone: 954-776-4456
E-mail: graduateschool@keiseruniversity.edu
Website: http://www.keiseruniversity.edu/graduateschool/PA/programs.php
Supplemental application: Yes, $50 fee
Number of students accepted into program each year: 25
Average GPA: >2.75
GRE: Yes
Length of program: 24 months
Uses CASPA: Yes
Tuition Cost: $50,000

Nova Southeastern University – Fort Lauderdale
Special focus: Primary Care
Location: Fort Lauderdale, FL
Degree granted: Master's Degree
Phone: 954-262-1109
E-mail: infopa@nsu.nova.edu
Website: http://www.nova.edu/pa/
Supplemental application: Yes, $50 fee
Number of students accepted into program each year: 75-80
Average GPA: 3.2
GRE: Yes
Length of program: 27 months
Uses CASPA: Yes
Tuition Cost: $68,397

Nova Southeastern University – Jacksonville
Special focus: Primary Care
Location: Jacksonville, FL
Degree granted: Master's Degree
Phone: 904-245-8990
E-mail: infopajex@nova.edu
Website: http://www.nova.edu/cah/pa/jacksonville/index.html
Supplemental application: Yes, $50 fee
Number of students accepted into program each year: 60
Average GPA: >2.9
GRE: Yes
Length of program: 27 months
Uses CASPA: Yes
Tuition Cost: $69,447

Nova Southeastern University – Orlando
Special focus: Primary Care
Location: Orlando, FL
Degree granted: Master's Degree
Phone: 407-264-5150
E-mail: pdyda@nova.edu
Website: http://www.nova.edu/cah/pa/orlando/index.html
Supplemental application: Yes, $50 fee
Number of students accepted into program each year: 60
Average GPA: >3.0
GRE: Yes
Length of program: 27 months
Uses CASPA: Yes
Tuition Cost: $67,697

Nova Southeastern University – Southwest Florida
Special focus: Primary Care
Location: Fort Myers, FL
Degree granted: Master's Degree
Phone: 954-262-1101 or 1-877-640-0218
E-mail: infopanaples@nsu.nova.edu
Website: http://www.nova.edu/cah/pa/swflorida/index.html
Supplemental application: Yes, $50 fee
Number of students accepted into program each year: 64
Average GPA: >2.9
GRE: Yes
Length of program: 27 months
Uses CASPA: Yes
Tuition Cost: $69,397

South University
Special focus: Primary Care
Location: Tampa, FL
Degree granted: Master's Degree
Phone: 813-393-3720
E-mail: paprogramtampa@southuniversity.edu
Website: http://www.abrandnewu.org/physician-assistant-program-
tampa.aspx?id=293&off
Supplemental application: No
Number of students accepted into program each year: 24
Average GPA: >2.6
GRE: Yes
Length of program: 27 months
Uses CASPA: Yes
Tuition Cost: $70,475

University of Florida
Special focus: Primary Care
Location: Gainesville, FL
Degree granted: Master's Degree
Phone: 352-265-7955
E-mail: cathleen.burdette@medicine.ufl.edu
Website: http://pap.med.ufl.edu/
Supplemental application: Yes
Number of students accepted into program each year: 60
Average GPA: 3.6
GRE: Yes
Length of program: 24 months
Uses CASPA: Yes
Tuition Cost: $55,940

Georgia

Emory University School of Medicine
Special focus: Primary Care
Location: Atlanta, GA
Degree granted: Master's Degree, Master of Public Health option available
Phone: 404-727-7857
E-mail: info@emorypa.org
Website: http://www.emorypa.org/
Supplemental application: Yes, $55 fee
Number of students accepted into program each year: 50
Average GPA: 3.4
GRE: Yes
Length of program: 28 month
Uses CASPA: Yes
Tuition Cost: $84,866

Georgia Health Sciences University
Special focus: Primary Care
Location: Augusta, GA
Degree granted: Master's Degree
Phone: 706-721-2725
E-mail: wpaschal@georgiahealth.edu
Website: http://www.georgiahealth.edu/sah/pa/
Supplemental application: Yes
Number of students accepted into program each year: 40
Average GPA: 3.4
GRE: Yes
Length of program: 27 months
Uses CASPA: No
Tuition Cost: $45,778 (in-state), $71,419 (out-of-state)

Mercer University College of Pharmacy and Health Sciences
Special focus: Primary Care
Location: Atlanta, GA
Degree granted: Master's Degree
Phone: 678-547-6232
E-mail: paprogram@mercer.edu
Website: http://cophs.mercer.edu/pa.htm
Supplemental application: Yes, $25 fee
Number of students accepted into program each year: 50
Average GPA: 3.4
GRE: Yes
Length of program: 28 months
Uses CASPA: Yes
Tuition Cost: $67,951

South University
Special focus: Primary Care
Location: Savannah, GA
Degree granted: Master's Degree
Phone: 912-201-8025
E-mail: susavadm@southuniversity.edu
Website: http://www.southuniversity.edu/physician-assistant-degree.aspx
Supplemental application: No
Number of students accepted into program each year: 65
Average GPA: >2.6
GRE: Yes
Length of program: 27 months
Uses CASPA: Yes
Tuition Cost: $64,345

Iowa

Des Moines University
Special focus: Primary Care
Location: Des Moines, IA
Degree granted: Master's Degree, Master of Public Health or Master of Health
Administration options available
Phone: 1-800-240-2767 ext. 7854
E-mail: paadmit@dmu.edu
Website: http://www.dmu.edu/pa/
Supplemental application: No
Number of students accepted into program each year: 50
Average GPA: 3.5
GRE: Yes
Length of program: 25 months
Uses CASPA: Yes
Tuition Cost: $55,571

University of Iowa
Special focus: Primary Care
Location: Iowa City, IA
Degree granted: Master's Degree
Phone: 319-335-8922
E-mail: paprogram@uiowa.edu
Website: http://paprogram.medicine.uiowa.edu/index.html
Supplemental application: No
Number of students accepted into program each year: 25
Average GPA: 3.7
GRE: Yes
Length of program: 25 months
Uses CASPA: Yes
Tuition Cost: $39,597 (in-state), $74,218 (out-of-state)

Idaho

Idaho State University
Special focus: Primary Care
Location: Pocatello, ID and Meridian, ID
Degree granted: Master's Degree
Phone: 208-282-4726
E-mail: pa@isu.edu
Website: http://www.isu.edu/PAprog/index.shtml
Supplemental application: Yes
Number of students accepted into program each year: 30 (Pocatello), and 30 (Meridian)
Average GPA: 3.8
GRE: Yes
Length of program: 24 months
Uses CASPA: Yes
Tuition Cost: $62,475 (in-state), $100,197 (out-of-state)

Illinois

Malcolm X College
Special focus: Primary Care
Location: Chicago, IL
Degree granted: Associate's Degree
Phone: 312-850-7255
E-mail: TKennon@ccc.edu
Website: http://malcolmx.ccc.edu/Academic_Programs/PhysicianAssistant.asp
Supplemental application: No
Number of students accepted into program each year: 26
Average GPA: >3.0
GRE: No
Length of program: 25 months
Uses CASPA: Yes
Tuition Cost: $11,147 (in-district), $24,684 (in-state), $29,114 (out-of-state)

Midwestern University
Special focus: Primary Care
Location: Downers Grove, IL
Degree granted: Master's Degree
Phone: 800-458-6253
E-mail: admissil@midwestern.edu
Website:
http://www.midwestern.edu/Programs_and_Admission/IL_Physician_Assistant_Studi
es.html Supplemental application: No
Number of students accepted into program each year: 86
Average GPA: 3.6
GRE: Yes
Length of program: 27 months
Uses CASPA: Yes
Tuition Cost: $80,325

Northwestern University
Special focus: Primary Care, Surgery, or Internal Medicine
Location: Chicago, IL
Degree granted: Master's Degree
Phone: 312-503-1851
E-mail: paprogram@northwestern.edu
Website: http://www.familymedicine.northwestern.edu/pa_program/
Supplemental application: Yes, $40
Number of students accepted into program each year: 30
Average GPA: 3.4
GRE: Yes
Length of program: 24 months
Uses CASPA: Yes
Tuition Cost: $75,423

Rosalind Franklin University of Medicine and Science
Special focus: Primary Care
Location: North Chicago, IL
Degree granted: Master's Degree
Phone: 847-589-8686
E-mail: pa.admissions@rosalindfranklin.edu
Website: http://www.rosalindfranklin.edu/dnn/CHP/PA/MS/tabid/1570/Default.aspx
Supplemental application: Yes, $35 fee
Number of students accepted into program each year: 60
Average GPA: >3.0
GRE: Yes
Length of program: 24 months
Uses CASPA: Yes
Tuition Cost: $61,520

Rush University
Special focus: Primary Care
Location: Chicago, IL
Degree granted: Master's Degree
Phone: 312-563-3234
E-mail: pa_admissions@rush.edu
Website:
http://www.rushu.rush.edu/servlet/Satellite?c=RushUnivLevel2Page&cid=125228377
0149&pagename=Rush/RushUnivLevel2Page/Level_2_College_GME_CME_Page
Supplemental application: Yes
Number of students accepted into program each year: 20
Average GPA: 3.3
GRE: Yes
Length of program: 33 months
Uses CASPA: Yes
Tuition Cost: $92,015

Southern Illinois University at Carbondale
Special focus: Primary Care
Location: Carbondale, IL
Degree granted: Master's Degree
Phone: 618-453-5527
E-mail: paadvisement-L@listserv.siu.edu
Website: http://paprogram.siuc.edu/
Supplemental application: Yes
Number of students accepted into program each year: 30
Average GPA: >3.0
GRE: Yes
Length of program: 26 months
Uses CASPA: No
Tuition Cost: $64,225 (in-state), $118,225 (out-of-state)

Indiana

Butler University/Clarian Health
Special focus: Primary Care
Location: Indianapolis, IN
Degree granted: Master's Degree, 5-year Freshman Entry Program option available
Phone: 317-940-9969
E-mail: dpearson@butler.edu or mliveret@butler.edu
Website: http://www.butler.edu/physician-assistant/
Supplemental application: No
Number of students accepted into program each year: 50
Average GPA: 3.4
GRE: No
Length of program: 30 months
Uses CASPA: Yes
Tuition Cost: $96,101

University of Saint Francis
Special focus: Primary Care
Location: Fort Wayne, IN
Degree granted: Master's Degree, BS/MS option available
Phone: 260-399-8000
E-mail: admis@sf.edu
Website: http://www.sf.edu/sf/physician-assistant
Supplemental application: No
Number of students accepted into program each year: 25
Average GPA: >3.0
GRE: Yes
Length of program: 27 months
Uses CASPA: Yes
Tuition Cost: $83,705

Kansas

Wichita State University
Special focus: Primary Care
Location: Wichita, KS
Degree granted: Master's Degree
Phone: 316-978-3011
E-mail: dee.mcdaniel@wichita.edu
Website: http://www.wichita.edu/pa
Supplemental application: Yes
Number of students accepted into program each year: 48 students
Average GPA: 3.6
GRE: No
Length of program: 26 months
Uses CASPA: Yes
Tuition Cost: $27,039 (in-state), $58,580 (out-of-state)

Kentucky

University of the Cumberlands
Special focus: Primary Care
Location: Williamsburg, KY
Degree granted: Master's Degree
Phone: 606-539-4398
E-mail: gradadm@ucumberlands.edu
Website: http://gradweb.ucumberlands.edu/medicine/mpas
Supplemental application: Yes
Number of students accepted into program each year: 20
Average GPA: >3.0
GRE: Yes
Length of program: 24 months
Uses CASPA: No
Tuition Cost: $64,511

University of Kentucky
Special focus: Primary Care
Location: Lexington, KY and Morehead, KY
Degree granted: Master's Degree
Phone: 859-323-1100
E-mail: gaboiss@uky.edu
Website: http://www.mc.uky.edu/PA/
Supplemental application: Yes
Number of students accepted into program each year: 40 (Lexington), and 16 (Morehead)
Average GPA: 3.4
GRE: Yes
Length of program: 29 months
Uses CASPA: Yes
Tuition Cost: $47,568 (in-state), $90,547 (out-of-state)

Louisiana

Louisiana State University Health Sciences Center
Special focus: Primary Care
Location: Shreveport, LA
Degree granted: Master's Degree
Phone: 318-813-2920
E-mail: kmeyer1@lsuhsc.edu
Website: http://www.medcom.lsuhscshreveport.edu/ah/
Supplemental application: No
Number of students accepted into program each year: 36
Average GPA: 3.5
GRE: Yes
Length of program: 27 months
Uses CASPA: Yes
Tuition Cost: $31,257 (in-state), $38,836 (out-of-state)

Our Lady of the Lake College
Special focus: Primary Care
Location: Baton Rouge, LA
Degree granted: Master's Degree
Phone: 225-768-1700
E-mail: andrea.williams@ololcollege.edu
Website: http://www.ololcollege-edu.org/content/admissions-academic-programs-physician-assistant-studies
Supplemental application: Yes
Number of students accepted into program each year: 30
Average GPA: 3.3
GRE: Yes
Length of program: 28 months
Uses CASPA: No
Tuition Cost: $84,376

Massachusetts

Massachusetts College of Pharmacy and Health Sciences – Boston
Special focus: Primary Care
Location: Boston, MA
Degree granted: Master's Degree
Phone: 617-732-2918
E-mail: paadmissions@mcphs.edu
Website: http://www.mcphs.edu/academics/programs/physician_assistant_studies/
Supplemental application: Yes
Number of students accepted into program each year: 75
Average GPA: 3.4
GRE: No
Length of program: 30 months
Uses CASPA: Yes
Tuition Cost: $95,375

Massachusetts College of Pharmacy and Health Sciences – Worcester
Special focus: Primary Care
Location: Worcester, MA
Degree granted: Master's Degree
Phone: 508-373-5607
E-mail: admissions.worcester@mcphs.edu
Website: http://www.mcphs.edu/academics/programs/physician_assistant_studies/
Supplemental application: Yes
Number of students accepted into program each year: 50
Average GPA: 3.4
GRE: No
Length of program: 24 months
Uses CASPA: Yes
Tuition Cost: $76,000

Northeastern University
Special focus: Primary Care
Location: Boston, MA
Degree granted: Master's Degree
Phone: 617-373-3195
E-mail: paprogram@neu.edu
Website: http://www.northeastern.edu//bouve/pa/
Supplemental application: Yes
Number of students accepted into program each year: 34-36
Average GPA: >3.0
GRE: No
Length of program: 24 months
Uses CASPA: Yes
Tuition Cost: $60,183

Springfield College
Special focus: Primary Care
Location: Springfield, MA
Degree granted: Master's Degree, 5-year BS/MS option
Phone: 413-748-3554
E-mail: glabelle@spfldcol.edu
Website: http://www.spfldcol.edu/
 Supplemental application: Yes
Number of students accepted into program each year: 30
Average GPA: >3.0
GRE: No
Length of program: 27 months
Uses CASPA: No
Tuition Cost: $93,600

Maryland

Anne Arundel Community College
Special focus: Primary Care
Location: Arnold, MD
Degree granted: Certificate, Master's Degree option
Phone: 410-777-7493
E-mail: ineun@aacc.edu or tdneall@aacc.edu
Website: http://www.aacc.edu/physassist/
Supplemental application: Yes
Number of students accepted into program each year: 40
Average GPA: 3.3
GRE: No
Length of program: 25 months
Uses CASPA: Yes
Tuition Cost: $19,226 (in-county), $27,407 (in-state), $40,537 (out-of-state)

Towson University – CCBC Essex
Special focus: Primary Care
Location: Baltimore, MD
Degree granted: Master's Degree
Phone: 410-704-4049
E-mail: mweinstein@towson.edu
Website: http://grad.towson.edu/program/master/past-ms/
Supplemental application: Yes
Number of students accepted into program each year: 35
Average GPA: 3.4
GRE: No
Length of program: 26 months
Uses CASPA: Yes
Tuition Cost: $22,716 (in-state), $47,268 (out-of-state)

University of Maryland – Eastern Shore
Special focus: Primary Care
Location: Princess Anne, MD
Degree granted: Bachelor's Degree
Phone: 410-651-7584
E-mail: padept@umes.edu
Website: http://www.umes.edu/PA/
Supplemental application: Yes
Number of students accepted into program each year: 35
Average GPA: >3.5
GRE: Yes
Length of program: 24 months
Uses CASPA: No
Tuition Cost: $22,893 (in-state), $44,151 (out-of-state)

Maine

The University of New England
Special focus: Primary Care
Location: Biddeford, ME
Degree granted: Master's Degree, 5-year BS/MS option
Phone: 207-221-4529
E-mail: admissions@une.edu
Website: http://www.une.edu/wchp/pa/
Supplemental application: No
Number of students accepted into program each year: 48-50
Average GPA: 3.5
GRE: No
Length of program: 24 months
Uses CASPA: Yes
Tuition Cost: $75,505

Michigan

Central Michigan University
Special focus: Primary Care
Location: Mount Pleasant, MI
Degree granted: Master's Degree
Phone: 989-774-1730
E-mail: chpadmit@cmich.edu
Website: http://www.cmich.edu/chp/x485.xml
Supplemental application: Yes
Number of students accepted into program each year: 40-45
Average GPA: 3.6
GRE: Yes
Length of program: 27 months
Uses CASPA: Yes
Tuition Cost: $60,172 (in-state), $94,892 (out-of-state)

Grand Valley State University
Special focus: Primary Care
Location: Grand Rapids, MI
Degree granted: Master's Degree
Phone: 616-331-3356
E-mail: zwartda@gvsu.edu
Website: http://www.gvsu.edu/pas/
Supplemental application: Yes
Number of students accepted into program each year: 32
Average GPA: 3.7
GRE: No
Length of program: 28 months
Uses CASPA: No
Tuition Cost: $49,815.00 (in-state), $67,911 (out-of-state)

University of Detroit Mercy
Special focus: Primary Care
Location: Detroit, MI
Degree granted: Master's Degree, 5-year BS/MS option, Part-time option
Phone: 313-993-1271
E-mail: chpgrad@udmercy.edu
Website: http://healthprofessions.udmercy.edu/programs/paprogram/pam/index.htm
Supplemental application: Yes
Number of students accepted into program each year: 30-40
Average GPA: 3.5
GRE: Yes
Length of program: 24 months or 36 months for Part-time option
Uses CASPA: Yes
Tuition Cost: $83,094

Wayne State University
Special focus: Primary Care
Location: Detroit, MI
Degree granted: Master's Degree
Phone: 313-577-1368
E-mail: paadmit@wayne.edu
Website: http://www.pa.cphs.wayne.edu/
Supplemental application: Yes
Number of students accepted into program each year: 48
Average GPA: >3.0
GRE: Yes
Length of program: 24 months
Uses CASPA: Yes
Tuition Cost: $37,817 (in-state), $67,606 (out-of-state)

Western Michigan University
Special focus: Primary Care
Location: Kalamazoo, MI
Degree granted: Master's Degree
Phone: 269-387-5311
E-mail: shannon.penny@wmich.edu
Website: http://www.wmich.edu/hhs/pa/
Supplemental application: No
Number of students accepted into program each year: 40
Average GPA: >3.0
GRE: No
Length of program: 24 months
Uses CASPA: Yes
Tuition Cost: $50,865 (in-state), $67,185 (out-of-state)

Minnesota

Augsburg College
Special focus: Primary Care
Location: Minneapolis, MN
Degree granted: Master's Degree
Phone: 612-330-1399
E-mail: paprog@augsburg.edu
Website: http://www.augsburg.edu/pa/
Supplemental application: Yes
Number of students accepted into program each year: 30
Average GPA: >3.0
GRE: No
Length of program: 36 months
Uses CASPA: Yes
Tuition Cost: $69,960

Mississippi

Mississippi College
Special focus: Primary Care
Location: Clinton, MS
Degree granted: Master's Degree
Phone: 601-925-7373
E-mail: lollar@mc.edu
Website: http://www.mc.edu/academics/departments/pa/
Supplemental application: No
Number of students accepted into program each year: 30
Average GPA: 3.5
GRE: Yes
Length of program: 30 months
Uses CASPA: Yes
Tuition Cost: $65,000

Missouri

Missouri State University
Special focus: Primary Care
Location: Springfield, MO
Degree granted: Master's Degree
Phone: 417-836-6151
E-mail: physicianasststudies@missouristate.edu
Website: http://www.missouristate.edu/pas/
Supplemental application: No
Number of students accepted into program each year: 30
Average GPA: 3.5
GRE: Yes
Length of program: 24 months
Uses CASPA: Yes
Tuition Cost: $20,916 (in-state), $39,757 (out-of-state)

Saint Louis University
Special focus: Primary Care
Location: St. Louis, MO
Degree granted: Master's Degree
Phone: 314-977-8521
E-mail: paprog@slu.edu
Website: http://www.slu.edu/x2348.xml
Supplemental application: Yes
Number of students accepted into program each year: 34
Average GPA: 3.5
GRE: No
Length of program: 27 months
Uses CASPA: Yes
Tuition Cost: $71,055

Montana

Rocky Mountain College
Special focus: Primary Care
Location: Billings, MT
Degree granted: Master's Degree
Phone: 406-657-1198
E-mail: pa@rocky.edu or pretlowm@rocky.edu
Website: http://www.rocky.edu/academics/programs/mpas/MPAS.shtml
Supplemental application: Yes
Number of students accepted into program each year: 34
Average GPA: >3.0
GRE: Yes
Length of program: 26 months
Uses CASPA: Yes
Tuition Cost: $88,717

North Carolina
Duke University Medical Center
Special focus: Primary Care
Location: Durham, NC
Degree granted: Master's Degree
Phone: 919-681-3155
E-mail: paadmission@mc.duke.edu
Website: http://pa.mc.duke.edu/
Supplemental application: Yes
Number of students accepted into program each year: 70
Average GPA: 3.4
GRE: Yes
Length of program: 24 months
Uses CASPA: Yes
Tuition Cost: $61,733

Campbell University
Special focus: Primary Care
Location: Buies Creek, NC
Degree granted: Master's Degree
Phone: 910-893-1690
E-mail: collettit@campbell.edu or pa@campbell.edu
Website: http://www.campbell.edu/paprogram
Supplemental application: Yes
Number of students accepted into program each year: 34
Average GPA: >3.2
GRE: Yes
Length of program: 28 months
Uses CASPA: Yes
Tuition Cost: $63,700

East Carolina University
Special focus: Primary Care
Location: Greenville, NC
Degree granted: Master's Degree
Phone: 252-744-1100
E-mail: pastudies@ecu.edu
Website: http://www.ecu.edu/pa/
Supplemental application: Yes
Number of students accepted into program each year: 33-35
Average GPA: 3.6
GRE: Yes
Length of program: 27 months
Uses CASPA: Yes
Tuition Cost: $10,955 (in-state), $48,359(out-of-state)

Methodist University
Special focus: Primary Care
Location: Fayetteville, NC
Degree granted: Master's Degree
Phone: 910-630-7495
E-mail: paprog@methodist.edu
Website: http://www.methodist.edu/paprogram/
Supplemental application: No
Number of students accepted into program each year: 40
Average GPA: 3.5
GRE: Yes
Length of program: 27 months
Uses CASPA: Yes
Tuition Cost: $67,900

Wake Forest University
Special focus: Primary Care
Location: Winston-Salem, NC
Degree granted: Master's Degree
Phone: 336-716-4356
E-mail: paadmit@wakehealth.edu
Website: http://www.wakehealth.edu/PAProgram/
Supplemental application: Yes
Number of students accepted into program each year: 64
Average GPA: 3.5
GRE: Yes
Length of program: 24 months
Uses CASPA: Yes
Tuition Cost: $53,127

Wingate University
Special focus: Primary Care
Location: Winston-Salem, NC
Degree granted: Master's Degree
Phone: (704) 233-8051
E-mail: pa@wingate.edu
Website: http://pa.wingate.edu/
Supplemental application: No
Number of students accepted into program each year: 33
Average GPA: 3.4
GRE: Yes
Length of program: 27 months
Uses CASPA: Yes
Tuition Cost: $66,679

North Dakota

University of North Dakota School of Medicine and Health Sciences
Special focus: Primary Care
Location: Grand Forks, ND
Degree granted: Master's Degree
Phone: 701-777-2491
E-mail: rhonda.mcdaniel@med.und.edu or paprogram@medicine.nodak.edu
Website: http://www.med.und.edu/physicianassistant/
Supplemental application: Yes
Number of students accepted into program each year: 70
Average GPA: >3.0
GRE: No
Length of program: 24 months
Uses CASPA: Yes
Tuition Cost: $41,505

Nebraska

Union College
Special focus: Primary Care
Location: Lincoln, NE
Degree granted: Master's Degree
Phone: 402-486-2527
E-mail: paprog@ucollege.edu
Website: http://www.ucollege.edu/pa
Supplemental application: No
Number of students accepted into program each year: 27
Average GPA: 3.3
GRE: No
Length of program: 32 months
Uses CASPA: Yes
Tuition Cost: $82,000

University of Nebraska Medical Center
Special focus: Primary Care
Location: Omaha, NE
Degree granted: Master's Degree
Phone: 402-559-6673
E-mail: sahpadmissions@unmc.edu
Website: http://www.unmc.edu/alliedhealth/pa/
Supplemental application: Yes
Number of students accepted into program each year: 42-44
Average GPA: 3.7
GRE: Yes
Length of program: 28 months
Uses CASPA: Yes
Tuition Cost: $33,794 (in-state), $91,143 (out-of-state)

New Hampshire

Franklin Pierce University
Special focus: Primary Care
Location: West Lebanon, NH
Degree granted: Master's Degree
Phone: 603-298-6617
E-mail: paprogram@franklinpierce.edu
Website:
http://www.franklinpierce.edu/academics/gradstudies/programs_of_study/master_phy
sician_assistant.htm Supplemental application: Yes
Number of students accepted into program each year: 24
Average GPA: >2.8
GRE: No
Length of program: 27 months
Uses CASPA: Yes
Tuition Cost: $86,016

Massachusetts College of Pharmacy and Health Sciences – Manchester
Special focus: Primary Care
Location: Manchester, NH
Degree granted: Master's Degree
Phone: 603-314-1763
E-mail: admissions@man.mcphs.edu or admissions.manchester@mcphs.edu
Website: http://www.mcphs.edu/academics/programs/physician_assistant_studies/
Supplemental application: Yes
Number of students accepted into program each year: 70
Average GPA: 3.4
GRE: No
Length of program: 24 months
Uses CASPA: Yes
Tuition Cost: $76,000

New Jersey

Seton Hall University
Special focus: Primary Care
Location: South Orange, NJ
Degree granted: Master's Degree
Phone: 973-275-2596
E-mail: joann.codella@shu.edu
Website: http://www.shu.edu/academics/gradmeded/ms-physician-assistant/index.cfm
Supplemental application: Yes
Number of students accepted into program each year: 30
Average GPA: >3.2
GRE: Yes
Length of program: 36 months
Uses CASPA: No
Tuition Cost: $90,816

University of Medicine and Dentistry of New Jersey
Special focus: Primary Care
Location: Piscataway, NJ
Degree granted: Master's Degree, BS/MS option, Public Health option, Part-time option
Phone: 732-235-4445
E-mail: shrpadm@umdnj.edu
Website: http://shrp.umdnj.edu/programs/paweb/index.html
Supplemental application: Yes
Number of students accepted into program each year: 50
Average GPA: 3.4
GRE: No
Length of program: 36 months
Uses CASPA: Yes
Tuition Cost: $64,365 (in-state), $91,520 (out-of-state)

New Mexico

The University of New Mexico School of Medicine
Special focus: Primary Care
Location: Albuquerque, NM
Degree granted: Master's Degree
Phone: 505-272-9864
E-mail: paprogram@salud.unm.edu
Website: http://hsc.unm.edu/som/fcm/pap/
Supplemental application: Yes
Number of students accepted into program each year: 16
Average GPA: 3.5
GRE: No
Length of program: 27 months
Uses CASPA: Yes
Tuition Cost: $22,302 (in-state), $50,863 (out-of-state)

University of St. Francis
Special focus: Primary Care
Location: Albuquerque, NM
Degree granted: Master's Degree
Phone: 888-446-4657
E-mail: aromero@stfrancis.edu
Website: http://www.stfrancis.edu/academics/college-of-arts-and-science/physician-assistant-studies/
Supplemental application: No
Number of students accepted into program each year: 34
Average GPA: >2.75
GRE: Yes
Length of program: 27 months
Uses CASPA: Yes
Tuition Cost: $ 62,064

Nevada

Touro University – Nevada
Special focus: Primary Care
Location: Henderson, NV
Degree granted: Master's Degree
Phone: 702-777-1750
E-mail: admissions@tun.touro.edu
Website: http://tun.touro.edu/programs/college-of-osteopathic-medicine/physician-assistant-studies/
Supplemental application: Yes
Number of students accepted into program each year: 56
Average GPA: >2.7
GRE: No
Length of program: 28 months
Uses CASPA: Yes
Tuition Cost: $75,383

New York

Albany Medical College
Special focus: Primary Care
Location: Albany, NY
Degree granted: Master's Degree
Phone: 518-262-5251
E-mail: greenr@mail.amc.edu
Website: http://www.amc.edu/Academic/PhysicianAssistant/index.html
Supplemental application: Yes
Number of students accepted into program each year: 40
Average GPA: 3.4
GRE: Yes
Length of program: 28 months
Uses CASPA: Yes
Tuition Cost: $47,243

Clarkson University
Special focus: Primary Care
Location: Potsdam, NY
Degree granted: Master's Degree
Phone: 315-268-7942
E-mail: pa@clarkson.edu
Website: http://www.clarkson.edu/pa/
Supplemental application: Yes
Number of students accepted into program each year: 15
Average GPA: >3.0
GRE: Yes
Length of program: 28 months
Uses CASPA: No
Tuition Cost: $82,500

Cornell University – Weill Medical College
Special focus: Surgical Care
Location: New York, NY
Degree granted: Master's Degree
Phone: 646-962-7277
E-mail: mshspa@med.cornell.edu
Website: http://www.med.cornell.edu/pa
Supplemental application: Yes
Number of students accepted into program each year: 32
Average GPA: 3.4
GRE: Yes
Length of program: 26 months
Uses CASPA: Yes
Tuition Cost: $76,761

CUNY York College
Special focus: Primary Care
Location: Jamaica, NY
Degree granted: Bachelor's Degree
Phone: 718-262-2823
E-mail: paprogram@york.cuny.edu
Website: http://www.york.cuny.edu/academics/departments/health-
professions/physician-assistant
Supplemental application: Yes
Number of students accepted into program each year: 30
Average GPA: >2.9
GRE: No
Length of program: 24 months
Uses CASPA: No
Tuition Cost: $17,415 (in-state), $23,370 (out-of-state)

The City College of New York / Sophie Davis School of Biomedical Education
Special focus: Primary Care
Location: New York, NY
Degree granted: Bachelor's Degree
Phone: 212-650-7745
E-mail: admissions@ccny.cuny.edu
Website: http://www1.ccny.cuny.edu/prospective/med/programs/paprogram.cfm
Supplemental application: Yes
Number of students accepted into program each year: 35
Average GPA: >2.5
GRE: No
Length of program: 28 months
Uses CASPA: No
Tuition Cost: $18,830 (in-state), $29,290 (out-of-state)

D'Youville College
Special focus: Primary Care
Location: Buffalo, NY
Degree granted: Master's Degree, optional BS/MS
Phone: 716-881-7713
E-mail: paprogram@dyc.edu
Website: http://www.dyc.edu/academics/physician_assistant/index.asp
Supplemental application: Yes
Number of students accepted into program each year: 40
Average GPA: 3.5
GRE: No
Length of program: 30 months
Uses CASPA: No
Tuition Cost: $74,746

Daemen College
Special focus: Primary Care
Location: Amherst, NY
Degree granted: Master's Degree, optional BS/MS
Phone: 716- 839-8383
E-mail: admissions@daemen.edu
Website:
http://www.daemen.edu/academics/divisionofhealthhumanservices/physicianassistant/
Pages/default.aspx
Supplemental application: No
Number of students accepted into program each year: 40
Average GPA: >3.0
GRE: No
Length of program: 33 months
Uses CASPA: Yes
Tuition Cost: $87,700

Hofstra University
Special focus: Primary Care
Location: Hempstead, NY
Degree granted: Master's Degree, optional BS/MS
Phone: 516-463-4074
E-mail: paprogram@hofstra.edu
Website: http://www.hofstra.edu/Academics/Colleges/HCLAS/PAP/
Supplemental application: Yes
Number of students accepted into program each year: 40
Average GPA: >3.0
GRE: No
Length of program: 28 months
Uses CASPA: Yes
Tuition Cost: $79,000

Le Moyne College
Special focus: Primary Care
Location: Syracuse, NY
Degree granted: Master's Degree, optional BS/MS
Phone: 315-445-4745
E-mail: PhysAssist@lemoyne.edu
Website: http://www.lemoyne.edu/tabid/654/Default.aspx
Supplemental application: Yes
Number of students accepted into program each year: 35-40
Average GPA: 3.2
GRE: No
Length of program: 24 months
Uses CASPA: Yes
Tuition Cost: $68,120

Long Island University
Special focus: Primary Care
Location: Brooklyn, NY
Degree granted: Master's Degree
Phone: 718-488-1011
E-mail: admissions@brooklyn.liu.edu
Website: http://www.liu.edu/Brooklyn/Academics/Schools/SHP/Dept/Physician-
Assistant/Graduate-Programs/MS-PAS.aspx
Supplemental application: Yes
Number of students accepted into program each year: 42
Average GPA: >3.0
GRE: Yes
Length of program: 28 months
Uses CASPA: Yes
Tuition Cost: $97,503

Mercy College
Special focus: Primary Care
Location: Bronx, NY
Degree granted: Master's Degree
Phone: 914-674-7635
E-mail: admissions@mercy.edu
Website: https://www.mercy.edu/academics/school-of-health-and-natural-
sciences/department-of-health-professions/ms-in-physician-assistant-studies/
Supplemental application: Yes
Number of students accepted into program each year: 40
Average GPA: 3.2
GRE: No
Length of program: 27 months
Uses CASPA: Yes
Tuition Cost: $82,400

New York Institute of Technology
Special focus: Primary Care
Location: Old Westbury, NY
Degree granted: Master's Degree, optional BS/MS
Phone: 516-686-3881
E-mail: pa@nyit.edu
Website: http://www.nyit.edu/physician_assistant_studies/
Supplemental application: No
Number of students accepted into program each year: 52
Average GPA: 3.3
GRE: Yes
Length of program: 30 months
Uses CASPA: Yes
Tuition Cost: $97,080

Pace University – Lenox Hill Hospital
Special focus: Primary Care
Location: New York, NY
Degree granted: Master's Degree
Phone: 212-346-1357
E-mail: paprogram@pace.edu
Website: http://www.pace.edu/lienhard/physician-assistant-studies/
Supplemental application: No
Number of students accepted into program each year: 50
Average GPA: >3.0
GRE: No
Length of program: 26 months
Uses CASPA: Yes
Tuition Cost: $82,833

Rochester Institute of Technology
Special focus: Primary Care
Location: Rochester, NY
Degree granted: Bachelor's Degree, optional BS/MS
Phone: 716-475-5151
E-mail: nhmscl@rit.edu
Website: http://www.rit.edu/cos/medical/physician_assistant.html
Supplemental application: Yes
Number of students accepted into program each year: 35-40
Average GPA: 3.0
GRE: No
Length of program: 21 months
Uses CASPA: No
Tuition Cost: $70,863

SUNY/Downstate Medical Center
Special focus: Primary Care
Location: Brooklyn, NY
Degree granted: Bachelor's Degree
Phone: 718-270-2325
E-mail: pa.chrp@downstate.edu
Website: http://www.downstate.edu/CHRP/pa/index.html
Supplemental application: Yes
Number of students accepted into program each year: 35
Average GPA: >2.75
GRE: No
Length of program: 27 months
Uses CASPA: No
Tuition Cost: $23,276 (in-state), $52,711 (out-of-state)

SUNY/Upstate Medical Center
Special focus: Primary Care
Location: Brooklyn, NY
Degree granted: Master's Degree
Phone: 315-464-6561
E-mail: admiss@upstate.edu
Website: www.upstate.edu/chp/programs/pa/
Supplemental application: Yes
Number of students accepted into program each year: 30
Average GPA: >3.0
GRE: Yes
Length of program: 27 months
Uses CASPA: Yes
Tuition Cost: $22,876 (in-state), $33,854 (out-of-state)

St. John's University
Special focus: Primary Care
Location: Fresh Meadows, NY
Degree granted: Bachelor's Degree
Phone: 718-990-8417
E-mail: admissions@stjohns.edu
Website: http://www.stjohns.edu/academics/undergraduate/pharmacy/programs/pa
Supplemental application: Yes
Number of students accepted into program each year: 75
Average GPA: >3.0
GRE: No
Length of program: 24 months
Uses CASPA: Yes
Tuition Cost: $73,205

Stony Brook University
Special focus: Primary Care
Location: Stony Brook, NY
Degree granted: Master's Degree
Phone: 631-444-3190
E-mail: paprogram@stonybrook.edu
Website: http://www.hsc.stonybrook.edu/shtm/pa/index.cfm
Supplemental application: Yes
Number of students accepted into program each year: 44
Average GPA: 3.2
GRE: No
Length of program: 24 months
Uses CASPA: Yes
Tuition Cost: $33,089 (in-state), $47,732 (out-of-state)

Touro College – Bay Shore
Special focus: Primary Care
Location: Bay Shore, NY
Degree granted: Master's Degree
Phone: 1-866-868-7648
E-mail: enrollhealth@touro.edu
Website: http://www1.touro.edu/shs/pali/pali.php
Supplemental application: Yes
Number of students accepted into program each year: 60
Average GPA: 3.3
GRE: No
Length of program: 24 months
Uses CASPA: Yes
Tuition Cost: $70,880

Touro College – Manhattan Campus
Special focus: Primary Care
Location: New York, NY
Degree granted: BS/MS
Phone: 212-463-0400, ext. 5792
E-mail: enrollhealth@touro.edu or astone@touro.edu
Website: http://www1.touro.edu/shs/pany/pany.php
Supplemental application: Yes
Number of students accepted into program each year: 35
Average GPA: 3.3
GRE: No
Length of program: 32 months (BS to MS)
Uses CASPA: Yes
Tuition Cost: $68,080

Wagner College
Special focus: Primary Care
Location: Staten Island, NY
Degree granted: BS/MS
Phone: 718-390-4151
E-mail: admissions@wagner.edu
Website: http://www.wagner.edu/departments/pa_program/
Supplemental application: Yes
Number of students accepted into program each year: 20
Average GPA: >3.0
GRE: No
Length of program: 36 months
Uses CASPA: No
Tuition Cost: $103,280

Ohio

Cuyahoga Community College / Cleveland State University
Special focus: Primary Care
Location: Cleveland, OH
Degree granted: Master's Degree
Phone: 216-987-5266
E-mail: Belinda.Wiggins@tri-c.edu
Website: http://www.tri-c.edu/programs/physicianassistant/Pages/default.aspx
Supplemental application: Yes
Number of students accepted into program each year: 35
Average GPA: >3.0
GRE: Yes
Length of program: 27 months
Uses CASPA: Yes
Tuition Cost: $30,000 (in-state), $46,977 (out-of-state)

Kettering College of Medical Arts
Special focus: Primary Care
Location: Kettering, OH
Degree granted: Master's Degree, optional BS/MS
Phone: 937-298-3399 ext. 55606
E-mail: PA@kcma.edu
Website: http://www.kcma.edu/Academics/PA/index.html
Supplemental application: No
Number of students accepted into program each year: 35-40
Average GPA: >3.0
GRE: No
Length of program: 27 months
Uses CASPA: Yes
Tuition Cost: $66,950

Marietta College
Special focus: Primary Care
Location: Marietta, OH
Degree granted: Master's Degree
Phone: 740-376-4458
E-mail: paprog@marietta.edu
Website: http://www.marietta.edu/departments/Physician_Assistant/index.html
Supplemental application: Yes
Number of students accepted into program each year: 36
Average GPA: 3.4
GRE: Yes
Length of program: 26 months
Uses CASPA: Yes
Tuition Cost: $70,904

The University of Findlay
Special focus: Primary Care
Location: Findlay, OH
Degree granted: Bachelor's Degree
Phone: 419-434-4529
E-mail: mcbride@findlay.edu
Website:
http://www.findlay.edu/academics/colleges/cohp/academicprograms/graduate/PHAS/
default.htm
Supplemental application: Yes
Number of students accepted into program each year: 18
Average GPA: 3.4
GRE: No
Length of program: 29 months
Uses CASPA: Yes
Tuition Cost: $78,060

University of Mount Union
Special focus: Primary Care
Location: Alliance, OH
Degree granted: Master's Degree
Phone: 1-800-334-6682
E-mail: scarpill@muc.edu
Website: http://www.mountunion.edu/pa
Supplemental application: Yes
Number of students accepted into program each year: 25-30
Average GPA: >3.0
GRE: Yes
Length of program: 27 month
Uses CASPA: Yes
Tuition Cost: $56,700

University of Toledo
Special focus: Primary Care
Location: Toledo, OH
Degree granted: Master's Degree
Phone: 419-383-3579
E-mail: grdsch@utnet.utoledo.edu
Website: http://www.utoledo.edu/med/grad/pa/index.html
Supplemental application: Yes
Number of students accepted into program each year: 40
Average GPA: >3.0
GRE: No
Length of program: 27 month
Uses CASPA: Yes
Tuition Cost: $51,553 (in-state), $82,284 (out-of-state)

Oklahoma

University of Oklahoma
Special focus: Primary Care
Location: Oklahoma City, OK
Degree granted: Master's Degree
Phone: 405-271-2058
E-mail: lillie-neal@ouhsc.edu
Website: http://www.ou.edu/content/tulsa/pa.html
Supplemental application: Yes
Number of students accepted into program each year: 50
Average GPA: 3.6
GRE: Yes
Length of program: 30 months
Uses CASPA: No
Tuition Cost: $44,440 (in-state), $74,528 (out-of-state)

University of Oklahoma – Tulsa
Special focus: Primary Care
Location: Tulsa, OK
Degree granted: Master's Degree
Phone: 918-619-4760
E-mail: tulsaweb@ouhsc.edu
Website: http://www.ou.edu/content/tulsa/pa.html
Supplemental application: Yes
Number of students accepted into program each year: 24
Average GPA: 3.5
GRE: Yes
Length of program: 30 months
Uses CASPA: No
Tuition Cost: $44,440 (in-state), $74,528 (out-of-state)

Oregon

Oregon Health Sciences University
Special focus: Primary Care
Location: Portland, OR
Degree granted: Master's Degree
Phone: 503-494-1484
E-mail: paprgm@ohsu.edu
Website: http://www.ohsu.edu/pa/
Supplemental application: Yes
Number of students accepted into program each year: 36
Average GPA: 3.5
GRE: Yes
Length of program: 26 months
Uses CASPA: Yes
Tuition Cost: $86,378

Pacific University
Special focus: Primary Care
Location: Forest Grove, OR
Degree granted: Master's Degree
Phone: 503-352-7272
E-mail: admissions@pacificu.edu
Website: http://www.pacificu.edu/pa/
Supplemental application: Yes
Number of students accepted into program each year: 44
Average GPA: 3.5
GRE: No
Length of program: 27 months
Uses CASPA: Yes
Tuition Cost: $79,011

Pennsylvania

Arcadia University
Special focus: Primary Care
Location: Glenside, PA
Degree granted: Master's Degree, optional Public Health program
Phone: 215-572-2910
E-mail: admiss@arcadia.edu
Website: http://www.arcadia.edu/academic/default.aspx?id=425
Supplemental application: No
Number of students accepted into program each year: 60
Average GPA: >3.2
GRE: Yes
Length of program: 24 months
Uses CASPA: Yes
Tuition Cost: $66,380

Chatham College
Special focus: Primary Care
Location: Pittsburgh, PA and San Juan, Puerto Rico
Degree granted: Master's Degree
Phone: 412-365-2988
E-mail: admissions@chatham.edu
Website: http://www.chatham.edu/departments/healthmgmt/graduate/pa/index.cfm
Supplemental application: No
Number of students accepted into program each year: 80
Average GPA: >3.0
GRE: No
Length of program: 24 months
Uses CASPA: Yes
Tuition Cost: $80,211

DeSales University
Special focus: Primary Care
Location: Center Valley, PA
Degree granted: Master's Degree, optional BS/MS
Phone: 610-282-1100 ext. 1415
E-mail: Linda.Schroeder@desales.edu
Website: http://www.desales.edu/default.aspx?pageid=331
Supplemental application: Yes
Number of students accepted into program each year: 40
Average GPA: 3.5
GRE: Yes
Length of program: 24 months
Uses CASPA: Yes
Tuition Cost: $66,636

Drexel University Hahnemann
Special focus: Primary Care
Location: Philadelphia, PA
Degree granted: Master's Degree
Phone: 215-762-4390
E-mail: js64@drexel.edu
Website: http://www.drexel.edu/physAsst/
Supplemental application: Yes
Number of students accepted into program each year: 75
Average GPA: >3.2
GRE: No
Length of program: 27 months
Uses CASPA: Yes
Tuition Cost: $76,610

Duquesne University
Special focus: Primary Care
Location: Pittsburgh, PA
Degree granted: Master's Degree (BS/MS degree program)
Phone: 412-396-6222
E-mail: tedrick@duq.edu
Website: http://www.duq.edu/physician-assistant/
Supplemental application: Yes
Number of students accepted into program each year: 35
Average GPA: >3.0
GRE: No
Length of program: 60 months
Uses CASPA: No
Tuition Cost: $152,232

Gannon University
Special focus: Primary Care
Location: Erie, PA
Degree granted: Master's Degree, optional BS/MS
Phone: 814-871-7606
E-mail: gillespi002@gannon.edu
Website: http://www.gannon.edu/departmental/pa/default.asp
Supplemental application: Yes
Number of students accepted into program each year: 48
Average GPA: >3.2
GRE: No
Length of program: 29 months
Uses CASPA: No
Tuition Cost: $90,690

Kings College
Special focus: Primary Care
Location: Wilkes-Barre, PA
Degree granted: Master's Degree, optional BS/MS
Phone: 570-208-5853
E-mail: Sharonkaminski@kings.edu
Website: http://departments.kings.edu/paprog/
Supplemental application: No
Number of students accepted into program each year: 45
Average GPA: >3.2
GRE: No
Length of program: 24 months
Uses CASPA: Yes
Tuition Cost: $70,858

Lock Haven University of Pennsylvania
Special focus: General
Location: Lock Haven, PA
Degree granted: Master's Degree, optional BS/MS
Phone: 570-484-2011
E-mail: gradadmissions@lhup.edu
Website: http://gradprograms.lhup.edu/pa/
Supplemental application: No
Number of students accepted into program each year: 70
Average GPA: >3.0
GRE: Yes
Length of program: 24 months
Uses CASPA: Yes
Tuition Cost: $34,278 (in-state), $50,184 (out-of-state)

Marywood University
Special focus: Primary Care, with option to specialize
Location: Scranton, PA
Degree granted: Master's Degree
Phone: 570-348-6298
E-mail: paprogram@marywood.edu
Website: http://www.marywood.edu/pa-program/
Supplemental application: No
Number of students accepted into program each year: 45
Average GPA: 3.0
GRE: Yes
Length of program: 27 months
Uses CASPA: Yes
Tuition Cost: $66,250

Pennsylvania College of Technology
Special focus: Primary Care
Location: Williamsport, PA
Degree granted: Bachelor's Degree
Phone: 570-320-2400
E-mail: kmayer@pct.edu
Website: http://www.pct.edu/schools/hs/pa/bpa.asp
Supplemental application: Yes
Number of students accepted into program each year: 30
Average GPA: >3.0
GRE: No
Length of program: 24 months
Uses CASPA: No
Tuition Cost: $47,000 (in-state), $57,798 (out-of-state)

Philadelphia College of Osteopathic Medicine
Special focus: Primary Care
Location: Philadelphia, PA
Degree granted: Master's Degree, optional BS/MS
Phone: 215-871-6700
E-mail: paadmissions@pcom.edu
Website:
http://www.pcom.edu/academic_programs/aca_pa/degree_programs_physician_assi/d
egree_programs_physician_assi.html
Supplemental application: Yes
Number of students accepted into program each year: 55
Average GPA: >3.0
GRE: No
Length of program: 26 months
Uses CASPA: Yes
Tuition Cost: $61,562

Philadelphia University
Special focus: Primary Care
Location: Philadelphia, PA
Degree granted: Master's Degree, optional BS/MS and optional MBA track
Phone: 215-951-2908
E-mail: gradadms@PhilaU.edu
Website: http://www.philau.edu/paprogram/
Supplemental application: Yes
Number of students accepted into program each year: 50
Average GPA: 3.3
GRE: Yes
Length of program: 25 months
Uses CASPA: Yes
Tuition Cost: $76,780

Salus University
Special focus: Primary Care
Location: Elkins Park, PA
Degree granted: Master's Degree
Phone: 215-780-1300 or 1-800-824-6262
E-mail: admissions@salus.edu
Website: http://www.salus.edu/physicianAssistant/index.html
Supplemental application: No
Number of students accepted into program each year: 32
Average GPA: 3.5
GRE: Yes
Length of program: 25 months
Uses CASPA: Yes
Tuition Cost: $65,645

Saint Francis University
Special focus: Primary Care
Location: Loretto, PA
Degree granted: Master's Degree, optional BS/MS
Phone: 814-472-3130
E-mail: pa@francis.edu
Website: http://www.francis.edu/MPAShome.htm
Supplemental application: No
Number of students accepted into program each year: 55-60
Average GPA: >3.0
GRE: No
Length of program: 24 months
Uses CASPA: Yes
Tuition Cost: $87,133

Seton Hill University
Special focus: Primary Care
Location: Greensburg, PA
Degree granted: Master's Degree, optional BS/MS
Phone: 724-838-4209
E-mail: lkomarny@setonhill.edu
Website: http://www.setonhill.edu/academics/pa/index.cfm
Supplemental application: No
Number of students accepted into program each year: 35
Average GPA: >3.2
GRE: No
Length of program: 27-29 months
Uses CASPA: Yes
Tuition Cost: $88,670

University of Pittsburgh
Special focus: Primary Care
Location: Pittsburgh, PA
Degree granted: Master's Degree
Phone: 412-624-6719
E-mail: admissions@shrs.pitt.edu
Website: http://www.shrs.pitt.edu/PA/
Supplemental application: Yes
Number of students accepted into program each year: 48
Average GPA: >3.0
GRE: Yes
Length of program: 24 months
Uses CASPA: Yes
Tuition Cost: $64,569 (in-state), $76,941 (out-of-state)

South Carolina

Medical University of South Carolina
Special focus: Primary Care
Location: Charleston, SC
Degree granted: Master's Degree
Phone: 843-792-3775
E-mail: longkk@musc.edu
Website: http://www.musc.edu/chp/pa/
Supplemental application: Yes
Number of students accepted into program each year: 65
Average GPA: >3.0
GRE: Yes
Length of program: 27 months
Uses CASPA: No
Tuition Cost: $70,253 (in-state), $102,431 (out-of-state)

South Dakota

University of South Dakota
Special focus: Primary Care
Location: Vermillion, SD
Degree granted: Master's Degree
Phone: 605-677-5128
E-mail: pa@usd.edu
Website: http://www.usd.edu/pa
Supplemental application: Yes
Number of students accepted into program each year: 20
Average GPA: 3.5
GRE: No
Length of program: 28 months
Uses CASPA: Yes
Tuition Cost: $46,777 (in-state), $81,825 (out-of-state)

Tennessee

Bethel College
Special focus: Primary Care
Location: McKenzie, TN
Degree granted: Master's Degree
Phone: (731) 352-4247
E-mail: hammondsk@bethelu.edu
Website: http://www.bethelu.edu/bethelpa/
Supplemental application: Yes
Number of students accepted into program each year: 36
Average GPA: 3.3
GRE: Yes
Length of program: 27 months
Uses CASPA: Yes
Tuition Cost: $61,250

Lincoln Memorial
Special focus: Primary Care
Location: Harrogate, TN
Degree granted: Master's Degree
Phone: (423)-869-6669
E-mail: PAAdmissions@lmunet.edu
Website: http://www.lmunet.edu/DCOM/pa/
Supplemental application: Yes
Number of students accepted into program each year: 80
Average GPA: >3.2
GRE: Yes
Length of program: 27 months
Uses CASPA: Yes
Tuition Cost: $67,474

South College
Special focus: Primary Care
Location: Knoxville, TN
Degree granted: Master's Degree
Phone: 865-251-1800
E-mail: pa_program@southcollegetn.edu
Website: http://www.southcollegetn.edu/masters/physician-assistant/
Supplemental application: Yes
Number of students accepted into program each year: 52
Average GPA: 3.0
GRE: Yes
Length of program: 27 months
Uses CASPA: Yes
Tuition Cost: $63,000

Trevecca Nazarene University
Special focus: Primary Care
Location: Nashville, TN
Degree granted: Master's Degree
Phone: 615-248-1225
E-mail: admissions_pa@trevecca.edu
Website: http://www.trevecca.edu/pa
Supplemental application: No
Number of students accepted into program each year: 48
Average GPA: >3.25
GRE: Yes
Length of program: 27 months
Uses CASPA: Yes
Tuition Cost: $72,964

Texas

Baylor College of Medicine
Special focus: Primary Care
Location: Houston, TX
Degree granted: Master's Degree
Phone: 713-798-4842
E-mail: admissions@bcm.edu
Website: http://www.bcm.edu/pap/
Supplemental application: Yes
Number of students accepted into program each year: 40
Average GPA: 3.5
GRE: Yes
Length of program: 30 months
Uses CASPA: Yes
Tuition Cost: $41,125

Interservice Physician Assistant Program
Special focus: Military Personnel Only
Location: Fort Sam Houston, TX
Degree granted: Master's Degree
Phone: 502-626-3735 ext. 60386
E-mail: ipap@usarec.army.mil
Website: http://www.usarec.army.mil/armypa/
Supplemental application: Yes
Number of students accepted into program each year: N/A
Average GPA: >3.0
GRE: No (SAT required instead)
Length of program: 36 months
Uses CASPA: No
Tuition Cost: N/A
(Note: Must be actively serving in order to qualify for admission)

Texas Tech University Health Sciences Center
Special focus: Primary Care
Location: Midland, TX
Degree granted: Master's Degree
Phone: 915-620-9905
E-mail: allied.health@ttuhsc.edu
Website: http://www.ttuhsc.edu/sah/mpa/
Supplemental application: Yes
Number of students accepted into program each year: 60
Average GPA: >3.2
GRE: No
Length of program: 27 months
Uses CASPA: Yes
Tuition Cost: $50,811 (in-state), or $89,561 (out-of-state)

University of North Texas
Special focus: Primary Care
Location: Fort Worth, TX
Degree granted: Master's Degree
Phone: 817-735-2003
E-mail: PAAdmissions@unthsc.edu
Website: http://www.hsc.unt.edu/education/pasp/
Supplemental application: Yes
Number of students accepted into program each year: 75
Average GPA: >3.0
GRE: Yes
Length of program: 34 months
Uses CASPA: Yes
Tuition Cost: $34,887 (in-state), $80,709 (out-of-state)

The University of Texas Health Science Center at San Antonio
Special focus: Primary Care
Location: San Antonio, TX
Degree granted: Master's Degree
Phone: 210-567-8744
E-mail: shpwelcome@uthscsa.edu
Website: http://www.uthscsa.edu/shp/pa/
Supplemental application: Yes
Number of students accepted into program each year: 30
Average GPA: 3.2
GRE: No
Length of program: 33 months
Uses CASPA: Yes
Tuition Cost: $27,989 (in-state), $78,000 (out-of-state)

The University of Texas Medical Branch at Galveston
Special focus: Primary Care
Location: Galveston, TX
Degree granted: Master's Degree
Phone: 409-772-3046
E-mail: PAS.web@utmb.edu
Website: http://www.sahs.utmb.edu/pas/
Supplemental application: Yes
Number of students accepted into program each year: 60
Average GPA: 3.6
GRE: Yes
Length of program: 26 months
Uses CASPA: Yes
Tuition Cost: $35,463 (in-state), $67,703 (out-of-state)

The University of Texas – Pan American
Special focus: Primary Care
Location: Edinburg, TX
Degree granted: Master's Degree
Phone: 956-381-2298
E-mail: pastudies@utpa.edu
Website: http://www.utpa.edu/dept/pasp/
Supplemental application: Yes
Number of students accepted into program each year: 25-40
Average GPA: 3.4
GRE: Yes
Length of program: 28 months
Uses CASPA: Yes
Tuition Cost: $35,652 (in-state), $62,632 (out-of-state)

University of Texas, Southwestern Medical Center at Dallas
Special focus: Primary Care
Location: Dallas, TX
Degree granted: Master's Degree
Phone: 214-648-1701
E-mail: pa.sshp@utsouthwestern.edu
Website: http://www.utsouthwestern.edu/utsw/cda/dept48945/files/54102.html
Supplemental application: No
Number of students accepted into program each year: 36
Average GPA: 3.7
GRE: Yes
Length of program: 31 months
Uses CASPA: Yes
Tuition Cost: $25,109 (in-state), $62,475 (out-of-state)

Utah

University of Utah
Special focus: Primary Care
Location: Salt Lake City, UT
Degree granted: Master's Degree
Phone: 801-581-7766
E-mail: admissions@upap.utah.edu
Website: http://web.utah.edu/upap/
Supplemental application: Yes
Number of students accepted into program each year: 40-44
Average GPA: 3.5
GRE: No
Length of program: 27 months
Uses CASPA: Yes
Tuition Cost: $55,319 (in-state), $82,225 (out-of-state)

Virginia

Eastern Virginia Medical School
Special focus: Primary Care
Location: Norfolk, VA
Degree granted: Master's Degree
Phone: 757-446-7158
E-mail: paprog@evms.edu
Website: http://www.evms.edu/evms-school-of-health-professions/physician-assistant.html
Supplemental application: Yes
Number of students accepted into program each year: 50
Average GPA: >3.0
GRE: No
Length of program: 27 months
Uses CASPA: Yes
Tuition Cost: $61,916 (in-state), $63,418 (out-of-state)

James Madison University
Special focus: Primary Care
Location: Harrisonburg, VA
Degree granted: Master's Degree
Phone: 540-568-2395
E-mail: paprogram@jmu.edu
Website: http://www.jmu.edu/healthsci/paweb/
Supplemental application: Yes
Number of students accepted into program each year: 25
Average GPA: 3.2
GRE: Yes
Length of program: 28 months
Uses CASPA: Yes
Tuition Cost: $28,554 (in-state), $78,366 (out-of-state)

Jefferson College of Health Sciences
Special focus: Primary Care
Location: Roanoke, VA
Degree granted: Master's Degree
Phone: 540-985-4016
E-mail: admissions@jchs.edu
Website: http://www.jchs.edu/page.php/prmID/382
Supplemental application: No
Number of students accepted into program each year: 40
Average GPA: 3.0
GRE: Yes
Length of program: 24 months
Uses CASPA: Yes
Tuition Cost: $68,215

Shenandoah University
Special focus: Primary Care
Location: Winchester, VA
Degree granted: Master's Degree
Phone: 540-542-6208
E-mail: pa@su.edu
Website: http://www.su.edu/pa/
Supplemental application: No
Number of students accepted into program each year: 38
Average GPA: 3.5
GRE: Yes
Length of program: 30 month
Uses CASPA: Yes
Tuition Cost: $64,328

Washington

University of Washington
Special focus: Primary Care
Location: Seattle, WA; Spokane, WA; Yakima, WA; and Anchorage, AK
Degree granted: Master's Degree, Bachelor's degree option
Phone: 206-616-4001
E-mail: medex@u.washington.edu
Website: http://www.washington.edu/medicine/som/depts/medex/
Supplemental application: Yes
Number of students accepted into program each year: 95-100
Average GPA: >3.0
GRE: Yes
Length of program: 27 months
Uses CASPA: Yes
Tuition Cost: $80,610

Washington DC

George Washington University
Special focus: Primary Care, with emphasis on Community Service
Location: Washington, DC
Degree granted: Master's Degree, Master of Public Health option available
Phone: 202-994-8528
E-mail: paadm@gwumc.edu or hsphora@gwu.edu
Website: http://www.gwumc.edu/healthsci/programs/pa/
Supplemental application: Yes, $60
Number of students accepted into program each year: 65
Average GPA: 3.4
GRE: Yes
Length of program: 24 months, or 36 months for MPH option
Uses CASPA: Yes
Tuition Cost: $77,765

Howard University
Special focus: Primary Care
Location: Washington, DC
Degree granted: Bachelor's Degree
Phone: 202-806-7536
E-mail: bdstephens@howard.edu or admission@howard.edu
Website: http://www.cpnahs.howard.edu/AHS/Pa/Introduction.htm
Supplemental application: Yes
Number of students accepted into program each year: 35
Average GPA: >2.8
GRE: No
Length of program: 26 months
Uses CASPA: Yes
Tuition Cost: $54,906

Wisconsin

Carroll University
Special focus: Primary Care
Location: Waukesha, WI
Degree granted: Master's Degree
Phone: 262-524-7643
E-mail: rharland@carrollu.edu
Website: http://www.carrollu.edu/gradprograms/physasst/default.asp
Supplemental application: Yes
Number of students accepted into program each year: N/A
Average GPA: >3.0
GRE: Yes
Length of program: 24 months
Uses CASPA: Yes
Tuition Cost: $54,582
GRE: Yes
Length of program: 24 months
Uses CASPA: Yes
Tuition Cost: $54,582

Marquette University
Special focus: Primary Care
Location: Milwaukee, WI
Degree granted: Master's Degree, Bachelor's degree option
Phone: 414-288-5688
E-mail: aubree.block@marquette.edu
Website: http://www.marquette.edu/chs/pa/index.shtml
Supplemental application: Yes
Number of students accepted into program each year: 50
Average GPA: 3.25
GRE: Yes
Length of program: 31 months
Uses CASPA: Yes
Tuition Cost: $91,230

University of Wisconsin – La Crosse
Special focus: Primary Care
Location: LaCrosse, WI
Degree granted: Master's Degree
Phone: 608-785-8470
E-mail: paprogram@uwlax.edu
Website: http://www.uwlax.edu/pastudies/
Supplemental application: Yes
Number of students accepted into program each year: 19
Average GPA: 3.7
GRE: Yes
Length of program: 24 months
Uses CASPA: Yes
Tuition Cost: $31,000 (in-state), $69,467 (out-of-state)

University of Wisconsin-Madison
Special focus: Primary Care
Location: Madison, WI
Degree granted: Master's Degree, part-time/distance options
Phone: 608-263-5620
E-mail: paprogram@mailplus.wisc.edu
Website: http://www.physicianassistant.wisc.edu/
Supplemental application: Yes
Number of students accepted into program each year: 36
Average GPA: >3.0
GRE: No
Length of program: 24 months
Uses CASPA: Yes
Tuition Cost: $37,140 (in-state), $76,388 (out-of-state)

West Virginia

Alderson Broaddus College
Special focus: Primary Care
Location: Philippi, WV
Degree granted: Master's Degree
Phone: 304-457-6256
E-mail: pa@ab.edu
Website: http://www.ab.edu/academics/master-science-physician-assistant-studies
Supplemental application: Yes
Number of students accepted into program each year: 36
Average GPA: >3.0
GRE: Yes
Length of program: 27 months
Uses CASPA: Yes
Tuition Cost: $84,000

Mountain State University
Special focus: Primary Care
Location: Beckley, WV
Degree granted: Master's Degree, and Bachelor's option
Phone: 304-92-1436
E-mail: ebrune@mountainstate.edu
Website:
http://www.mountainstate.edu/majors/onlinecatalogs/graduate/programs/PhysiciansA
ssistant.aspx
Supplemental application: Yes
Number of students accepted into program each year: 50
Average GPA: 3.0
GRE: No
Length of program: 34 months
Uses CASPA: No
Tuition Cost: $67,855

International PA Programs

James Cook University, Townsville, Australia
Website: http://www.jcu.edu.au/

Prince Sultan Military College of Health Sciences, Saudi Arabia
Website http://www.psmchs.edu.sa/index.php/departments/42

Birmingham University, United Kingdom
Website: http://www.medicine.bham.ac.uk/pg/assistant/docs/appguidance0910.pdf

St. George's University of London, United Kingdom
Website: http://www.sgul.ac.uk/postgraduate/taught-courses/postgraduate-diploma-
physician-assistant-studies-1

University of Wolverhamptom, United Kingdom
Website: http://www.wlv.ac.uk/default.aspx?page=17177

Index of Residencies and Fellowship Programs

Below, you will find a list of the current PA residencies and fellowships. However, as information frequently changes, I urge you to review the list online at http://www.appap.org. You will notice that only a handful of the programs are currently accredited, as accreditation for postgraduate programs is optional.

(It is important to keep in mind that some of the programs that are not currently accredited are currently undergoing the process to become accredited)

Acute Care Medicine

- University of Missouri; Columbia, MO
  Contact Person: Terry Carlisle
  Phone: 573-882-0808
  E-mail: Carlislet@health.missouri.edu
  Website: http://www.medicine.missouri.edu/acutepa/

Cardiology

- University of Illinois; Rockford, IL
  Contact Person: Tina Kaatz
  Phone: 815-395-5858
  E-mail: tkaatz@uic.edu
  Website:
  http://www.rockford.medicine.uic.edu/cms/one.aspx?objectId=4916065&contextId=515172

Cardiothoracic Surgery

- The Methodist DeBakey Heart Center; Houston, TX
  Contact Person: Boris Bratovich
  Phone: 713-441-6201 or 713-790-2089
  E-mail: borisbratovich@sbcglobal.net
  Website: http://www.methodisthealth.com/mcsa.cfm?id=35343

- North Shore University Hospital; Manhasset, NY
  Contact Person: Robert Blenderman
  Phone: 516-562-4489
  E-mail: Rblender@nshs.edu

- St. Joseph Mercy Hospital; Ypsilanti, MI
  Contact Person: Scott A. Rogers
  Phone: 734-712-5418
  E-mail: rogerssc@trinity-health.org
  Website: http://www.stjoeshealth.org/PhysicianAssistantResidencyProgram

- Emory Physician Assistant Postgraduate Cardiothoracic Surgical Residency
  Program; Atlanta, GA
  Contact Person: Christopher Nickum
  Phone: (404) 686-2513
  E-mail: christopher.nickum@emoryhealthcare.org
  Website: http://www.surgery.emory.edu/divisions/cardiothoracic-
  surgery/PA_postgrad_cardio_residency.html

Critical Care

- Johns Hopkins Hospital; Baltimore, MD
  Contact Person: Brad Winters
  Phone: 410-502-2651
  E-mail: paccres@jhmi.edu
  Website:
  http://www.hopkinsmedicine.org/surgery/education/pacc_residency/index.ht
  ml

- Oregon Health and Sciences University, Portland, OR
  Contact Person: Amy Juve
  Phone: 503-494-7641
  E-mail: juvea@ohsu.edu
  Website: http://www.ohsu.edu/anesth/recruitment/PA.htm

- Winthrop University Hospital; Mineola, NY
  Contact person: Frizzuto@winthrop.org
  Phone: 516-663-9278
  E-mail: Frank Rizzuto
  Website: http://www.winthrop.org/departments/education/physician-
  assistant-postgraduate-surgical-critical-care-residency-training/

- University of Massachusetts Medical Center; Worcester, MA
  Contact Person: Christina Bailey
  Phone: 774-443-7552
  E-mail: baileyc@ummhc.org

- Montefiore Medical Center; Bronx, NY
  Contact Person: David Keith
  Phone: 718-920-8442
  E-mail: dkeith@montefiore.org
  Website:
  http://www.einstein.yu.edu/medicine/criticalcare/critical_education.aspx?id=
  21583&bid=21582&ekmensel=15074e5e_870_3206_btnlink

- The Methodist Hospital Physician Organization; Houston, TX
  Contact Person: Kamlesh Thaker
  Phone: 713-441-3620
  E-mail: kthaker@tmhs.org or gowens@tmhs.org

Dermatology

- Center for Dermatology and Dermatologic Surgery; Washington, DC
  Contact Person: Cheryl Burgess
  Phone: 202-955-5757
  E-mail: PAFP@ct4dermatology.com

Emergency Medicine

- Johns Hopkins Bayview Medical Center; Baltimore, MD
  Contact Person: Jonathan Lerner
  Phone: 410-550-7911
  E-mail: paerres@jhmi.edu
  Website: http://www.hopkinsbayview.org/emresidency/index.html

- United States Army – Baylor University; Fort Sam Houston, TX
  Contact Person: Major Sue Love
  Phone: 210-916-4542
  E-mail: sue.love@us.army.mil
  Website: http://www.baylor.edu/graduate/index.php?id=51996

- Arrowhead Regional medical Center; Colton, CA
  Contact Person: Nicole Silva
  Phone: 909-580-2175
  E-mail: silva@armc.sbcounty.gov
  Website: http://www.empafellowship.com

- University of Iowa; Iowa City, IA
  Contact Person: Mark Nunge
  Phone: 319-384-6511
  E-mail: mark-nunge@uiowa.edu
  Website:
  http://www.healthcare.uiowa.edu/EmergencyMedicine/paResidency.html

- Staten Island University Hospital; Staten Island, NY
  Contact Person: Bartholomew Cambria
  Phone: 718-226-1492
  E-mail: bcambria@siuh.edu

- Bassett Medical Center; Cooperstown, NY
  Contact Person: Kevin Kinkade
  Phone: 607-547-4762
  E-mail: Kevin.Kinkade@bassett.org
  Website: http://www.bassett.org/bassett-medical-center/medical-
  education/residency-programs/rural-emergency-medicine-postgraduate-
  physician-assistant-program/

- New York Presbyterian Hospital; New York, NY
  Contact Person: Rahul Sharma
  Phone: 212-746-0780
  E-mail: Sharma@med.cornell.edu
  Website: http://web.me.com/brooks16pa/Cornell_EMPA/Home.html

- Albert Einstein Medical Center; Philadelphia, PA
  Contact Person: Lynn Scherer
  Phone: 215-456-1956
  E-mail: SchererL@einstein.edu
  Website: http://www.einstein.edu/education/programs/38-pi/em-physician-
  assistant.html

- Marquette University Aurora Health Care; Milwaukee, WI
  Contact Person: Mary Jo Wiemiller
  Phone: 414-288-5688
  E-mail: maryjo.wiemiller@marquette.edu

Hospitalist

- Mayo Clinic Arizona, Phoenix, Arizona
  Contact Person: Kristen Will or Zachary Hartsell
  Phone: 480-342-1387
  E-mail: will.kristen@mayo.edu or hartsell.zachary@mayo.edu
  Website: http://www.mayo.edu/mshs/pa-him-sct.html
  *Currently Accredited

Neonatology

1. University of Kentucky; Lexington, KY
   Contact Person: Eric Reynolds
   Phone: 859-323-5530
   E-mail: ereyn2@uky.edu
   Website: http://ukhealthcare.uky.edu/KCH/education/neonatalresidency.asp

Nephrology

- University of Illinois; Rockford, IL
  Contact Person: Tina Kaatz
  Phone: 815-395-5858
  E-mail: tkaatz@uic.edu
  Website: http://www.rockfordnephrology.org/

- Rosalind Franklin University; North Chicago, IL
  Contact Person: Walter Falkowski
  Phone: 847-578-3000
  E-mail: bchnning@nmua.info

Neurosurgery

- University of Arizona; Tucson, AZ
  Contact Person: Julie Schippers or Martin Weinand
  Phone: 520-626-0704
  E-mail: julies@u.arizona.edu or mweinand@email.arizona.edu

- Geisinger Medical Center; Danville, PA
  Contact Person: Anupama Bedi
  Phone: 570-214-9265
  E-mail: abedi1@geisinger.edu

- Texas Brain and Spine Institute; Bryan, TX
  Contact Person: Joe Hlavin
  Phone: 979-204-3103
  E-mail: jhlavi@txbsi.com
  Website: http://www.ctxeg.org/

Ob-Gyn

- Riverside-Arrowhead Regional Medical Center; Colton, CA
  Contact Person: Christine Sims
  Phone: 909-580-6320
  E-mail: Simsch@armc.sbcounty.gov
  Website: http://temp.obgynpanet.officelive.com/default.aspx

- Montefiore Medical Center; Bronx, NY
  Contact Person: Jose Lopez
  Phone: 718-781-9644
  E-mail: jlopez@montefiore.org

Oncology

- MD Anderson Cancer Center; Houston, TX
  Contact Person: Maura Polansky
  Phone: 713-794-5002
  E-mail: mpolansk@mdanderson.org
  *Currently Accredited

Orthopaedic Surgery

- Arrowhead Regional Medical Center; Colton, CA
  Contact Person: Julie Mabry
  Phone: 909-580-6353/6330
  E-mail: N/A
  Currently Accredited

- Illinois Bone and Joint Institute; Park Ridge, IL
  Contact Person: Patrick Knott
  Phone: 847-578-8689
  E-mail: patrick.knott@rosalindfranklin.edu
  Website:
  http://www.rosalindfranklin.edu/dnn/chp/home/chp/pa/orthopaedicresidency.
  aspx

- NYU Hospital for Joint Diseases; New York, NY
  Contact Person: Steven DeBrocky
  Phone: 212-598-2339
  E-mail: steven.debrocky@nyumc.org

- Watauga Orthopedics; Johnson City, TN
  Contact Person: Robert Rogan
  Phone: (423) 282-9011
  E-mail: roganrb@wtodocs.com
  Website: www.Wataugaortho.com

- Naval Medical Center (Portsmouth)
  *Currently Accredited

- University of Illinois; Rockford, IL
  Contact Person: Tina Kaatz
  Phone: 815-395-5858
  E-mail: tkaatz@uic.edu
  Website: http://www.rockfordortho.com/physicians/fellowships.html

Otolaryngology

- Mayo Clinic; Phoenix, AZ
  Contact Person: John Stroh
  Phone: 480-342-2983
  E-mail: stroh.john@mayo.edu
  Website: http://www.mayo.edu/mshs/pa-otorhino-sct.html

Psychiatry

- Cherokee Mental Health Institute; Cherokee, IA
  Contact Person: Daniel W. Gillette
  Phone: 712-225-2594
  E-mail: dgillet@dhs.state.ia.us
  Website: http://www.psychiatricpa.com/

- Regions Hospital; St. Paul, MN
  Contact Person: Tracy Keizer
  Phone: 651-254-1563
  E-mail: Tracy.b.keizer@healthpartners.com

- University of Iowa Behavioral Health; Iowa City, IA
  Contact Person: Michael Flaum
  Phone: 319-353-4340
  E-mail: michael-flaum@uiowa.edu
  Website: http://www.uihealthcare.com/depts/med/psychiatry/residents/

Surgery

- Arrowhead Regional Medical Center; Colton, CA
  Contact Person: Victor Joe
  Phone: 909-580-6210
  E-mail: joev@armc.sbcounty.gov

- Bassett Healthcare; Cooperstown, NY
  Contact Person: Shari Johnson-Ploutz
  Phone: 607-547-3202
  E-mail: shari.johnson-ploutz@bassett.org
  Website: http://www.bassett.org/bassett-medical-center/medical-education/

- Duke University Medical Center; Durham, NC
  Contact Person: Sherry Davi
  Phone: 919-681-7891
  E-mail: sherry.davi@duke.edu
  Website: http://general.surgery.duke.edu/education-and-training/residency-programs/pa-surgical-residency-program
  *Currently Accredited

- Grand Rapids Medical Education and Research Center; Grand Rapids, MI
  Contact Person: Kristen Norris
  Phone: 616-391-8651
  E-mail: pasrp@spectrum-health.org

- The Johns Hopkins Hospital; Baltimore, MD
  Contact Person: Barish Edil
  Phone: 410-502-2651
  E-mail: pasurgres@jhmi.edu
  Website:
  http://www.hopkinsmedicine.org/surgery/education/pa_residency/index.html
  *Currently Accredited

- Montefiore Medical Center, Bronx, NY
  Contact Person: Robert Sammartano
  Phone: 718-920-6223
  E-mail: rsammart@montefiore.org

- The Hospital of Central Connecticut; New Britain, CT
  Contact Person: Richard L. Commaille
  Phone: 860-224-5513
  E-mail: rcommail@thocc.org
  Website: http://www.thocc.org/physicians/pasurgicalresidency.aspx

- Norwalk Hospital/Yale University of Medicine; Norwalk, CT
  Contact Person: Virginia O. Hilton
  Phone: 203-852-2188
  E-mail: ginny.hilton@norwalkhealth.org
  Website: http://www.norwalkhospital.org/common.aspx?id=2559

- Medical College of Wisconsin; Milwaukee, WI
  Contact Person: Kim Somers
  Phone: 414-266-6593
  E-mail: surgeryed@mcw.edu
  Website: http://www.mcw.edu/pgpaprogram.htm

Trauma/Critical Care

- Bridgeport Hospital, Bridgeport, CT
  Contact Person: Paul Possenti
  Phone: 203-384-4213
  E-mail: ppposs@bpthospital.org

- St. Luke's Hospital; Bethlehem, PA

Contact Person: Laurie N. Wilson
Phone: 610-954-2207
E-mail: wilsonla@slhn.org

- Wake Med Health and Hospitals; Raleigh, NC
  Contact Person: Gloria Garver
  Phone: 919-350-8729
  E-mail: Ggarver@wakemed.org

- Intermountain Medical Center; Murray, UT
  Contact Person: Mary Ruth Pugh
  Phone: 801-507-6556
  E-mail: mary.pugh2@imail.org

Urology

- University of Illinois; Rockford, IL
  Contact Person: Tina Kaatz
  Phone: 815-395-5858
  E-mail: tkaatz@uic.edu
  Website:
  http://www.rockford.medicine.uic.edu/cms/one.aspx?objectId=4916065&contextId=515172

- University of Texas Southwestern at Dallas; Dallas, TX
  Contact Person: Brad Hornberger
  Phone: 214-645-9765
  E-mail: Brad.Hornberger@UTSouthwestern.edu
  Website:
  http://www.utsouthwestern.edu/utsw/cda/dept10803/files/605079.html

Teaching Fellowships

- Medical University of South Carolina; Charleston, SC
  Contact Person: Kelly Long
  Phone: 843-792-3775
  E-mail: longkk@musc.edu
  Website: http://academicdepartments.musc.edu/chp/pa/fellow.htm

- Duke University Medical Center; Durham, NC
  Contact Person: Karen J. Hills
  Phone: 919-668-6400
  E-mail: karen.hills@duke.edu
  Website: http://paprogram.mc.duke.edu/Post-Graduate/Teaching-Fellowship/

- Rosalind Franklin University; North Chicago, IL
  Contact Person: Patrick Knott
  Phone: 847-578-8302
  E-mail: Patrick.Knott@RosalindFranklin.edu
  Website:
  http://www.rosalindfranklin.edu/dnn/CHP/PA/Fellowship/tabid/1575/Default.aspx

Index of Physician Assistant Professional Organizations

There are many physician assistant organizations, caucuses, and special interest groups. Additionally, each state has its own PA-specific chapter. You should also seek further information by visiting the AAPA website (that information is listed below).

These specialty organizations are currently recognized by the AAPA:

The American Academy of Physician Assistants ("AAPA")
Website: http://www.aapa.org
Content: AAPA is the organization created by PAs for PAs. This website has everything you will want to know about becoming a PA and being a PA.

The Physician Assistant Education Association ("PAEA")
Website: http://www.paeaonline.org
Content: PAEA is the only organization that specifically represents Physician Assistant educational programs.

The American Association of Surgical Physician Assistants ("AASPA")
Website: http://www.aaspa.com
Content: AASPA is the premiere multi-specialty organization for PAs, PA students, and pre-PA students interested in surgery.

The Society of Emergency Medicine Physician Assistants ("SEMPA")
Website: http://www.sempa.org/
Content: SEMPA represents emergency medicine PAs in the United States and around the world.

Physician Assistants in Orthopaedic Surgery ("PAOS")
Website: http://www.paos.org
Content: PAOS is the national organization that represents Physician Assistants in orthopaedics and in all orthopaedic employment settings. Its membership also includes Physician Assistant students and supporters of the profession.

The Association of Physician Assistants in Cardiovascular Surgery ("APACVS")
Website: http://www.apacvs.org
Content: APACVS is the premiere organization representing the interests of Cardiovascular and Thoracic Surgical Physician Assistants.

The Association of Neurosurgical Physician Assistants ("ANSPA")
Website: http://www.anspa.org
Content: ANSPA is dedicated to the promotion and development of Physician Assistants working in Neurological Surgery.

Society of Dermatology Physician Assistants
Website: http://www.dermpa.org
Content: The Society of Dermatology Physician Assistants promotes the interests of PAs and students in dermatology.

Society of Physician Assistants in Otorhinolaryngology / Head & Neck Surgery ("ENTPA")
Website: http://www.entpa.org
Content: ENTPA promotes the growth and development of Physician Assistants in the ENT field.

American Academy of Nephrology Physician Assistants ("AANPA")
Website: http://www.aanpa.org
Content: AANPA supports the professional growth, development, training, education and networking of PAs within the specialty practice of nephrology.

American Academy of Physician Assistants in Occupational Medicine
Website: http://www.aapaoccmed.org
Content: American Academy of Physician Assistants in Occupational Medicine is an educational organization representing PAs who share a common interest and role in the care of the working person, and the prevention of workplace illness and injury.

American Society of Endocrine Physician Assistants
Website: http://www.endocrine-pa.com
Content: The American Society of Endocrine Physician Assistants is dedicated to the education, advancement and placement of PAs in endocrinology.

Association of Physician Assistants in Cardiology
Website: http://cardiologypa.org
Content: The Association of Physician Assistants in Cardiology is a resource for cardiology PAs and PA students.

Association of Physician Assistants in Obstetrics & Gynecology ("PAOBGYN")
Website: http://www.paobgyn.org
Content: PAOBGYN is the only professional association devoted exclusively to PAs practicing in women's health.

Association of Physician Assistants in Oncology ("APAO")
Website: http://www.apao.cc
Content: APAO promotes the utilization of Physician Assistants in the delivery of the best possible care available to people with cancer and related diseases.

Association of Physician Assistants in Anesthesia
Website: http://www.anesthesiapa.org
Content: The Association of Physician Assistants in Anesthesia serves as a resource for PAs working in anesthesia.

Association of Plastic Surgery Physician Assistants ("APSPA")
Website: http://www.apspa.net
Content: APSPA serves PAs and students interested in working in plastic surgery.

Association of Psychiatric Physician Assistants
Website: http://www.psychpa.org
Content: The Association of Psychiatric Physician Assistants is dedicated to Physician Assistants who work in the area of mental health care.

Society for Physician Assistants in Pediatrics
Website: http://www.spaponline.org
Content: The Society for Physician Assistants in Pediatrics consists of PAs, PA residents and PA students, as well as affiliate and associate individuals who share a common interest in the art of pediatric medicine.

Society of Physician Assistants Caring for the Elderly
Website: http://www.geri-pa.org
Content: The Society of Physician Assistants Caring for the Elderly shares information about practicing geriatric medicine as it relates to Physician Assistants and other health care providers.

Society of Physician Assistants in Rheumatology
Website: http://www.rheumpas.org
Content: The Society of Physician Assistants in Rheumatology enhances the health and well being of persons with Rheumatological disorders through the representation and advancement of PA/physician teams.

Association of Family Practice Physician Assistants ("AFPPA")
Website: http://www.afppa.org
Content: AFPPA is the only national organization representing primary care Physician Assistants.

Gastroenterology Physician Assistants
Website: http://www.gipas.org
Content: The Gastroenterology Physician Assistants organization is the voice representing Physician Assistants who practice in Gastroenterology and Hepatology.

Urological Association of Physician Assistants
Website: http://www.uapanet.org
Content: The Urological Association of Physician Assistants supports the advancement of physician assistants in urology.

Military and Government PA Organizations:

Veteran Affairs Physician Assistant Association
Website: http://www.vapaa.org
Content: The Veteran Affairs Physician Assistant Association promotes the interests of Physician Assistants employed by the U.S. Department of Veterans Affairs.

Society of Air Force Physician Assistants
Website: http://www.safpa.org
Content: The Society of Air Force Physician Assistants is dedicated to PAs who work in the Air Force community.

Naval Association of Physician Assistants
Website: http://www.aapa.org/napa
Content: The Naval Association of Physician Assistants is devoted to educating the public about the PA profession, seeking legislative and governmental policy changes regarding PAs, and informing those in the profession about national Navy issues.

The Society of Army Physician Assistants
Website: http://www.sapa.org
Content: A civilian organization representing and supporting U.S. Army Physician Assistants, including former, active, retired, reserve and National Guard PAs.

International PA Organizations:

United Kingdom Association of Physician Assistants ("UKAPA")
Website: http://www.ukapa.co.uk
Content: The UK Association of Physician Assistants supports the PA profession in the United Kingdom.

Index

Made in the USA
Lexington, KY
15 June 2012